Tuberculosis Control
in the WHO
Western Pacific Region

2003 Report

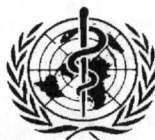

World Health Organization
Office for the Western Pacific Region

Acknowledgements

We would like to thank all tuberculosis managers and statisticians from all the countries and areas of the Western Pacific Region for providing data for this publication.

WHO Library Cataloguing in Publication Data

Tuberculosis Control in the WHO Western Pacific Region : 2003 report

1. Tuberculosis — epidemiology. 2. Western Pacific

ISBN 92 9061 043 3   (NLM Classification: WF 205)

Contents

Acknowledgements   ii

Abbreviations   v

Map: Tuberculosis situation in the Western Pacific Region (all types), 2001   vi

Summary   vii

Table 1: Key indicators of tuberculosis control in the Western Pacific Region, 2001   viii

Part I: Commentary   1

Chapter 1
Review of tuberculosis epidemiology   2

Chapter 2
Review of DOTS implementation and treatment results   7

Chapter 3
Tuberculosis control in high-burden countries   10

Part II: Tables   15

Table 5   Notification of tuberculosis cases by type, Western Pacific Region, 2001   17

Table 6   Age and sex distribution of new sputum smear-positive cases in
           DOTS and non-DOTS areas, Western Pacific Region, 2001   18

Table 7   Notification rate per 100 000 of new smear-positive cases by age
           and sex in DOTS and non-DOTS areas, Western Pacific Region, 2001   19

Table 8   Trend in notified tuberculosis cases (all types) in DOTS and non-DOTS areas   20

Table 9   Trend in notified cases (new smear-positives) in DOTS and
           non-DOTS areas   21

Table 10   Trend in tuberculosis notification rates per 100 000 population (all types)   22

Table 11   Trend in tuberculosis notification rates per 100 000 population
           (smear-positives)   23

Table 12   Trend in tuberculosis notification (number of all types) in DOTS and
           non-DOTS areas, 1998–2001   24

Table 13   Trend in tuberculosis notification (number of new smear-positives) in DOTS
           and non-DOTS areas, 1998–2001   24

Table 14   Trend in tuberculosis notification (rate for all types) in DOTS and
           non-DOTS areas, 1998–2001   26

Table 15   Trend in tuberculosis notification (rate for new smear-positives) in DOTS
           and non-DOTS areas, 1998–2001   26

Table 16   Treatment outcome of new smear-positive cases registered in 2000
           in DOTS areas   28

Contents

Table 17 Treatment outcome of new smear-positive cases registered in 2000
         in non-DOTS areas   29
Table 18 Treatment outcome of re-treatment cases registered in 2000 in
         DOTS areas   30
Table 19 Treatment outcome of re-treatment cases registered in 2000 in
         non-DOTS areas   31

Part III: Charts   33
Chart 1 Notification of all cases (rate per 100 000) by country, Western Pacific
         Region, 2001   34
Chart 2 Notification of new smear-positive cases (rate per 100 000) by country,
         Western Pacific Region, 2001   35
Chart 3 Notification rate of new smear-positive cases by age and sex in DOTS
         areas, Western Pacific Region, 2001   36
Chart 4 DOTS enrolment rate in high-burden countries, Western Pacific Region,
         2001   36
Chart 5 DOTS enrolment rate of new smear-positive cases in high-burden
         countries, Western Pacific Region, 1997 and 2001   37
Chart 6 DOTS case detection rate of new smear-positive cases in high-burden
         countries, Western Pacific Region, 2001   37
Chart 7 Treatment success of new smear-positive cases under DOTS in high-
         burden countries, Western Pacific Region, 2001   38
Chart 8 DOTS progress in high-burden countries in the Western Pacific Region,
         1998–2001   38

Annexes   39
Annex 1 Profiles of high-burden countries in the Western Pacific Region   40
Annex 2 Definitions   48

Abbreviations

AFB   Acid Fast Bacilli
DOT   Directly Observed Treatment
DOTS   Directly Observed Treatment Short-Course
HIV   Human Immunodeficiency Virus
NTP   National Tuberculosis Programme
TB   Tuberculosis
WHO   World Health Organization
WPR   Western Pacific Region (of WHO)

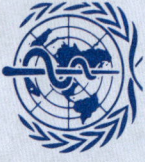

World Health Organization
Regional Office for the Western Pacific

Tuberculosis Situation in the Western Pacific Region (All Types), 2001

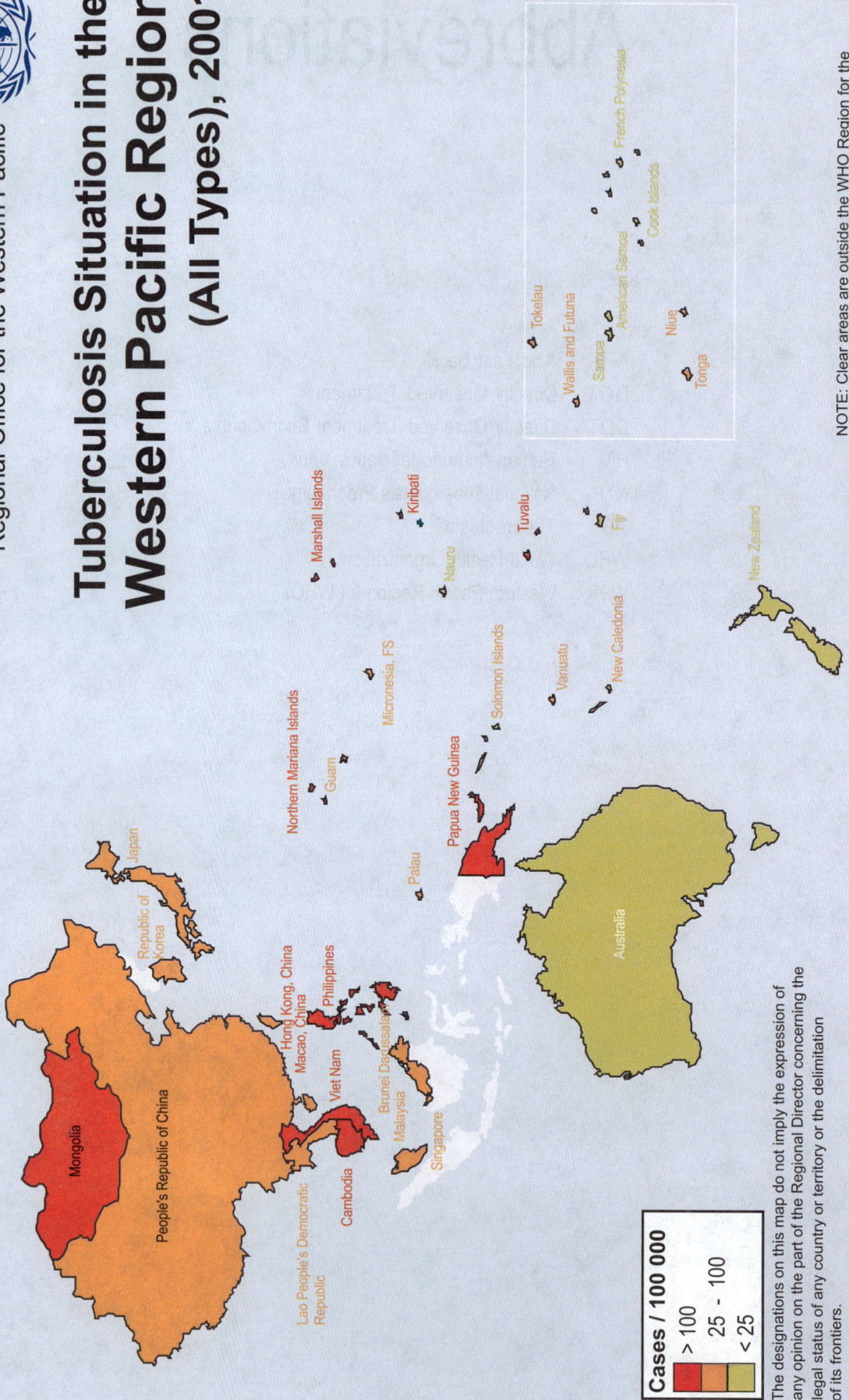

Cases / 100 000

- > 100
- 25 - 100
- < 25

The designations on this map do not imply the expression of any opinion on the part of the Regional Director concerning the legal status of any country or territory or the delimitation of its frontiers.

Pacific islands not to scale.

NOTE: Clear areas are outside the WHO Region for the Western Pacific.

Mongolia

People's Republic of China

Japan

Republic of Korea

Hong Kong, China

Macao, China

Viet Nam

Philippines

Lao People's Democratic Republic

Cambodia

Brunei Darussalam

Malaysia

Singapore

Northern Mariana Islands

Guam

Palau

Marshall Islands

Kiribati

Nauru

Micronesia, FS

Tuvalu

Fiji

Papua New Guinea

Solomon Islands

Vanuatu

New Caledonia

Australia

New Zealand

Tokelau

Wallis and Futuna

Samoa

American Samoa

French Polynesia

Cook Islands

Niue

Tonga

Summary

This 2003 report is an update on the epidemiological situation of tuberculosis in the Western Pacific Region and shows the progress of Directly Observed Treatment Short-course (DOTS) programmes. National Tuberculosis Programmes of 33 countries and areas (accounting for a total population of 1.702 billion[1]) submitted data on cases notified during 2001 and the treatment results of the cohort of patients registered during 2000. A standard form was used, based on common definitions and variables.

In 2001, the 33 countries and areas notified 811 263 tuberculosis cases (all types) and 379 060 new smear-positive pulmonary cases. Notification rates were 48 per 100 000 and 22 per 100 000, respectively, showing no significant variation from recent years (Table 1, page viii). About 69% of the notified tuberculosis patients were aged 15–54, which is the most productive age group, while the group aged 25–34 had the highest tuberculosis burden at 20% (all cases) (Table 6, page 18).

Based on the estimated incidence for 2001, the case detection rate was 40% for all types and 41% for smear-positive cases (Table 1), well short of the World Health Organization (WHO) target of 70%. Higher case detection rates were observed in DOTS areas (31% for all types and 37% for new smear-positive cases) compared to non-DOTS areas (9% and 5%, respectively) (Table 1). Further DOTS expansion should lead to an increase in case detection, especially of the most contagious cases – those that are pulmonary smear-positive.

About 68% of the regional population had access to DOTS. The DOTS enrolment rate for new smear-positive cases increased to 89%, from 78% in 2000 (Table 1). The treatment success rate was 92.3% (Table 16, page 28) for pulmonary new smear-positive patients registered in 2000. Out of these, 89% were cured, exceeding the WHO target of 85%.

Among the seven countries with the highest burden of tuberculosis in the Region (Cambodia, the People's Republic of China, the Lao People's Democratic Republic, Mongolia, Papua New Guinea, the Philippines, and Viet Nam) Mongolia and Viet Nam passed WHO targets of 70% DOTS case detection and 85% treatment success (for new smear-positive cases). Mongolia passed the WHO targets during 2001, two years after full DOTS coverage was achieved in 1999. The Philippines, although not yet reaching the target for detection (57% in 2001), managed almost full DOTS coverage, five years after the introduction of DOTS.

In some countries, an increase was seen in the number of human immunodeficiency virus (HIV) patients with tuberculosis. For instance, HIV prevalence among tuberculosis patients increased from 6% in 2000 to 8.4% in 2002 in Cambodia (see profiles of high-burden countries in Annex 1). The level of primary multidrug resistance in China is also a cause for concern.

> In 2001, the 33 countries and areas notified 811 263 tuberculosis cases (all types) and 379 060 new smear-positive pulmonary cases.

---

[1] Population update 2001, Global Tuberculosis Control, WHO, Geneva.

TABLE 1

Key indicators of tuberculosis control in the Western Pacific Region, 2001

Country	*Pop. x 1000	Notification in DOTS and non-DOTS areas — All cases Number	All cases Rate	New S+ Number	New S+ Rate	New S+ %	*No. of estimated cases All cases	*No. of estimated cases New S+	Case detection rate All cases (%)	Case detection rate New S+ (%)	Pop. with access to DOTS Pop.	Pop. with access to DOTS %	No. of cases in DOTS areas All cases	No. of cases in DOTS areas New S+	No. of cases in non-DOTS areas All cases	No. of cases in non-DOTS areas New S+	**DOTS enrolment rate All cases (%)	**DOTS enrolment rate New S+ (%)	***DOTS case detection rate All cases (%)	***DOTS case detection rate New S+ (%)	Non-DOTS case detection rate All cases (%)	Non-DOTS case detection rate New S+ (%)
	a	b	c	d	e	f=d/b	g	h	i=b/g	j=d/h	k	l	m	n	o	p	q=m/b	r=n/d	s=m/g	t=n/h	u=o/g	v=p/h
American Samoa	70	3	4	2	3	67	23	11	13	19	70	100	0	0	3	2	0	0	0	0	13	19
Australia	19 338	980	5	228	1	23	1528	687	64	33	10 443	54	485	99	495	129	49	43	32	14	32	19
Brunei Darussalam	335	216	65	95	28	44	185	83	116	114	335	100	216	95	0	0	100	100	116	114	0	0
Cambodia	13 441	19 170	143	14 361	107	75	78 564	35 118	24	41	13 441	100	19 170	14 361	0	0	100	100	24	41	0	0
China	1 284 972	485 221	38	212 766	17	44	1 447 947	651 110	34	33	873 781	68	362 172	188 480	123 049	24 286	75	89	25	29	8	4
Cook Islands	20	2	10	2	10	100	7	3	30	67	20	100	2	2	0	0	100	100	30	67	0	0
Fiji	823	183	22	73	9	40	276	124	66	59	823	100	183	73	0	0	100	100	66	59	0	0
French Polynesia	237	45	19	24	10	53	80	36	56	67	230	97	45	24	0	0	100	100	56	67	0	0
Guam	158	63	40	47	30	75	133	60	47	78	158	100	63	47	0	0	100	100	47	78	0	0
Hong Kong, China	6961	7262	104	1853	27	26	5755	2587	126	72	6961	100	5907	1425	1355	428	81	77	103	55	24	17
Japan	127 335	35 489	28	11 408	9	32	44 954	20 227	79	56	58 574	46	17 809	5709	17 680	5699	50	50	40	28	39	28
Kiribati	84	189	225	64	76	34	71	32	267	201	84	100	189	64	0	0	100	100	267	201	0	0
Republic of Korea	47 069	37 268	79	11 805	25	32	32 787	14 721	114	80	0	0	0	0	37 268	11 805	0	0	0	0	114	80
Lao PDR	5403	2382	44	1533	28	64	12 789	5755	19	27	4323	80	1618	1533	764	0	68	100	13	27	6	6
Macao, China	449	465	104	157	35	34	371	167	125	94	449	100	465	157	0	0	100	100	125	94	0	0
Malaysia	22 633	14 830	66	8309	37	56	27 119	12 149	55	68	22 633	100	14 830	8309	0	0	100	100	55	68	0	0
N. Mariana Islands	76	58	76	19	25	33	64	29	91	66	76	100	58	19	0	0	100	100	91	66	0	0
Marshall Islands	52	56	108	15	29	27	44	20	128	76	52	100	56	15	0	0	100	100	128	76	0	0
Micronesia, FS	126	95	75	8	6	8	106	48	90	17	88	70	95	8	0	0	100	100	90	17	0	0
Mongolia	2559	3526	138	1631	64	46	5041	2268	70	72	2559	100	3526	1631	0	0	100	100	70	72	0	0
Nauru	13	3	24	2	16	67	4	2	71	106	13	100	3	2	0	0	100	100	71	106	0	0
New Caledonia	220	64	29	34	15	53	185	83	35	41	0	0	0	0	64	34	0	0	0	0	35	41
New Zealand	3808	377	10	68	2	18	409	184	92	37	3808	100	89	21	288	47	24	31	22	11	70	26
Niue	2	0	0	0	0	0	1	0	0	0	2	100	0	0	0	0	0	0	0	0	0	0
Palau	20	0	0	0	0	0	17	7	0	0	13	100	0	0	0	0	0	0	0	0	0	0
Papua New Guinea	4920	3470	71	462	9	13	11 771	5285	29	9	640	13	3470	462	0	0	100	100	29	9	0	0
Philippines	77 131	107 133	139	59 341	77	55	232 266	104 439	46	57	74 817	97	107 133	59 341	0	0	100	100	46	57	0	0
Pitcairn Islands	0																					
Samoa	159	22	14	12	8	55	53	24	41	50	159	100	22	12	0	0	100	100	41	50	0	0
Singapore	4108	1536	37	357	9	23	1874	842	82	42	4108	100	749	175	787	182	49	49	40	21	42	22
Solomon Islands	463	292	63	118	25	40	390	176	75	67	417	90	292	118	0	0	100	100	75	67	0	0
Tokelau	1	0	0	0	0	0	0	0	0	0	0	0	0	0	0	0	0	0	0	0	0	0
Tonga	99	11	11	8	8	73	33	15	33	53	97	98	11	8	0	0	100	100	33	53	0	0
Tuvalu	10	0	0	0	0	0	3	2	0	0	0	0	0	0	0	0	0	0	0	0	0	0
Vanuatu	202	173	86	56	28	32	170	77	102	73	131	65	121	46	52	10	70	82	71	60	31	13
Viet Nam	79 175	90 679	115	54 202	68	60	143 412	64 535	63	84	79 016	100	90 679	54 202	0	0	100	100	63	84	31	0
Wallis and Futuna	15	0	0	0	0	0	5	2	0	0												
Western Pacific	1 702 484	811 263	47.7	379 060	22.3	47	2 048 439	920 908	40	41	1 158 305	68	629 458	336 438	181 805	42 622	78	89	31	37	9	5

* 2001 update, WHO Geneva.

** DOTS enrolment rate is the proportion of all detected cases that are diagnosed and treated in DOTS areas.

*** DOTS detection rate is the proportion of total estimated cases that are diagnosed and treated under DOTS.

PART I
Commentary

Chapter 1
Review of tuberculosis epidemiology   2

Chapter 2
Review of DOTS implementation and treatment results   7

Chapter 3
Tuberculosis control in high-burden countries   10

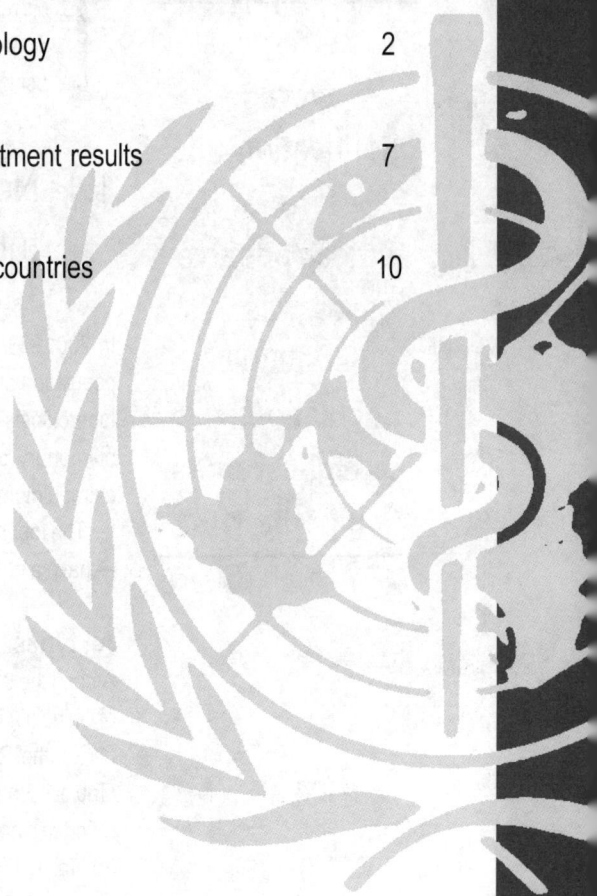

Commentary

Review of tuberculosis epidemiology

The regional average notification rate for new smear-positive cases was 22.3 per 100 000 population, with the highest rate in Cambodia (107).

This report is based on case notification and treatment outcome data supplied by National Tuberculosis Programmes (NTPs) to the World Health Organization (WHO) for 2001, using a standard data collection form, with common definitions and variables.

1.1 Notification of tuberculosis cases by type of tuberculosis

In 2001, 33 out of 37 countries and areas of the Western Pacific Region with a combined population of 1.702 billion submitted tuberculosis data for 2001. Together, they notified 811 263 tuberculosis cases (all types[2]) (47.7 per 100 000 population), 379 060 new smear-positive pulmonary cases (22.3 per 100 000), 307 228 new pulmonary smear-negatives, 32 852 extrapulmonary cases and 36 178 relapses (Tables 1, page viii, and 5, page 17).

The four non-reporting countries – Palau, the Pitcairn Islands, Tuvalu, and Wallis and Fortuna — have a combined population of only 45 000.

All types

Among the 811 263 tuberculosis cases (all types) in the Region (Figure 1), the People's Republic of China (China) notified 485 221 cases (61%), the Philippines 107 133 (13%), Viet Nam 90 679 (11%), the Republic of Korea 37 268 (5%), Japan 35 489 (4%) and Cambodia 19 170 (2%) (Table 1, Page viii). The 27 other countries together notified 36 303 cases (4%). Eight countries reported a notification rate (all types) greater than 100, and 13 countries reported a rate lower than 30 (Table 1).

Pulmonary new smear-positive cases

Out of the 379 060 new smear-positive cases in the Region, China notified 212 766 cases (56%), the Philippines 59 341 (16%), Viet Nam 54 202 (14%), Cambodia 14 361 (4%), Korea 11 805 (3%) and Japan 11 408 (3%). The 27 other countries together notified 15 177 cases (4%) (Tables 1 and 5).

The regional average notification rate for new smear-positive cases was 22.3 per 100 000 population, with the highest rate in Cambodia (107). The rate ranged between 25 and 100 in 15 countries: 77 in the Philippines; 76 in Kiribati; 68 in Viet Nam; 64 in Mongolia; 37 in

---

[2] In 2001, 956 re-treatment after failure cases and 23 667 other re-treatment cases were not included in the notification.

FIGURE 1

Distribution of notified tuberculosis all types by country, Western Pacific Region, 2001

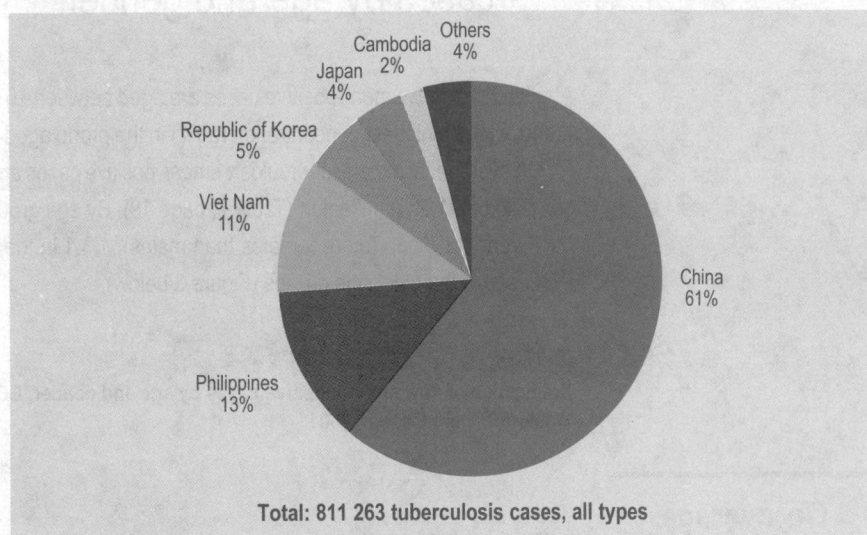

Total: 811 263 tuberculosis cases, all types

Malaysia; 35 in Macao, China; 30 in Guam; 29 in the Marshall Islands; 28 in Brunei Darussalam, the Lao People's Democratic Republic and Vanuatu; 27 in Hong Kong, China; and 25 in the Republic of Korea, the Northern Mariana Islands and Solomon Islands. China notified 17 new smear-positive cases per 100 000 population. Four industrialized countries (Japan, Australia, New Zealand and Singapore) and 12 Pacific island countries had lower rates (Table 1, page viii).

The proportion of new smear-positive cases out of all notified cases was 47% for the Region. China's rate was 44%. Thirteen countries, including five of the seven with the highest burden (Cambodia, the Lao People's Democratic Republic, Mongolia, the Philippines and Viet Nam) notified proportions higher than 50% (Table 1).

Directly Observed Treatment Short-course (DOTS) areas reported 53% of new smear-positive cases (336 438 new smear-positives out of 629 458 all cases) compared to only 23% in non-DOTS areas (42 622 new smear-positives out of 181 805 all cases) (Table 1 and Figure 2).

Extrapulmonary tuberculosis cases were not reported in China. The 32 852 extrapulmonary cases reported in the 32 other countries represented 4% of all notified cases (Table 5, page 17).

FIGURE 2

Notified cases by type of tuberculosis in DOTS and non-DOTS areas, Western Pacific Region, 2001

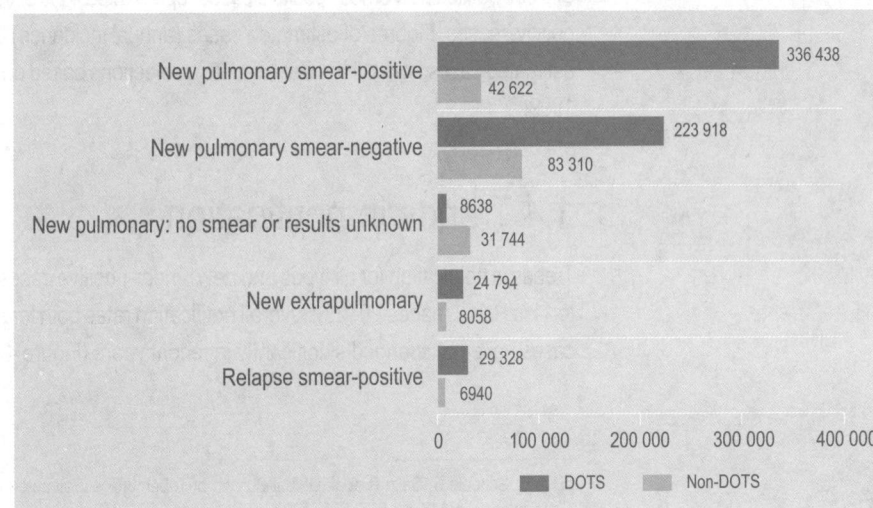

1.2 Notification of new smear-positive pulmonary cases by age and gender

About 69% of new smear-positive cases are aged between 15 and 54, the most productive age group, with the highest concentration (20%) in the group aged 25–34 (Table 6, page 18).

On average, two male tuberculosis smear-positive cases are notified for every female one (a sex ratio of 2:1) in the Region (Table 7, page 19). By age group, the sex ratio was 0.8:1 in the 0–14 year old group (more females than males), 1.3:1 in the 15–24 year old group and then increased in the older age groups (Figure 3 below).

FIGURE 3

Notification of new smear-positive cases by age and gender, DOTS and non-DOTS areas, Western Pacific Region, 2001

> On average, two male tuberculosis smear-positive cases are notified for every female one (a sex ratio of 2:1) in the Region.

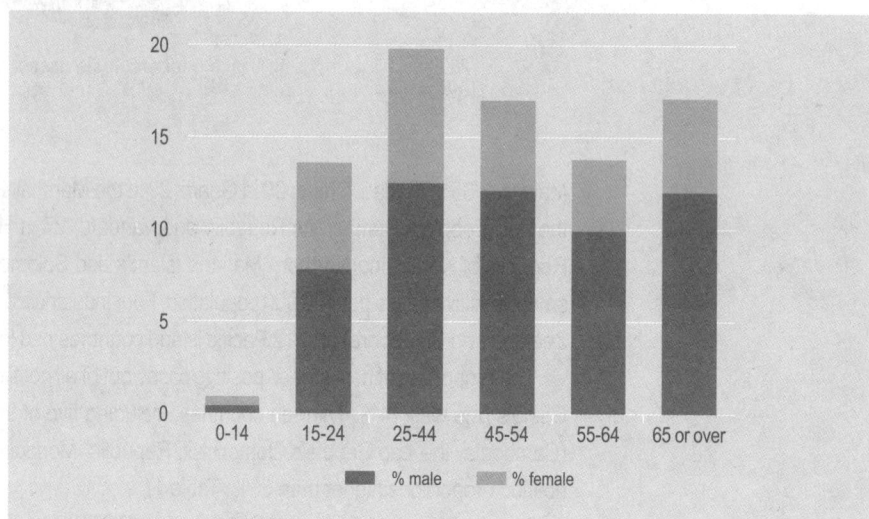

1.3 Case detection rate

The case detection rate (see Annex 2 for definition) was 40% for all tuberculosis cases and 41% for new smear-positive cases (Table 1, page viii). In other words, in the Region, the 811 263 notified cases (all types) represented 40% of the 2 048 439 estimated cases (all types) and the 379 060 notified new smear-positive cases represented 41% of the 920 908 estimated new smear-positive cases. Figures of estimated cases (annual incidence) are based on the 2001 update of estimated cases from WHO, Geneva, with projections based on *Global Burden of Tuberculosis*,[3] 1999.

1.4 Trends in notification

Trends in notification for all types and new smear-positive cases are given by country in Tables 8 to 11 in Part II (pages 20–23). Overall notification rates both for all types and new smear-positive cases have not changed significantly in recent years (Figure 4 opposite). Trends in notification

---

[3] Dye C, Scheele S, Dalin P et al. Global Burden of Tuberculosis. Estimated Incidence, Prevalence, and Mortality by Country. JAMA 282: 677–686, 1999.

may reflect variations in performance in case finding as well as changes in the burden of the disease. They may thus be misleading, with their interpretation biased by variations in the reporting system and/or the use of different denominators (estimates of population). Moreover, trends in case detection rates will also be affected by changes in the estimated incidence.

FIGURE 4

Trend in notification rates of tuberculosis, Western Pacific Region, 1993–2001

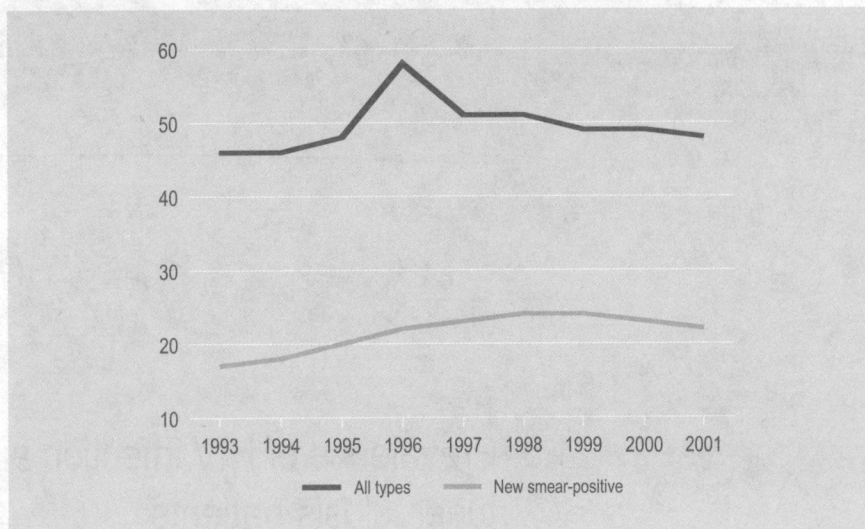

For individual countries, notification increased slightly in China and Viet Nam after 1998, but decreased in Cambodia and the Philippines (Table 2, below, and Figure 5, overleaf).

TABLE 2

Trend in case notification (rates per 100 000) in Cambodia, China, the Philippines and Viet Nam, Western Pacific Region, 1995–2001

	1995	1996	1997	1998	1999	2000	2001
Cambodia							
All	146	145	149	158	175	157	143
New S +	111	117	121	129	143	123	107
China							
All	29	38	34	36	36	37	38
New S +	11	14	15	17	17	17	17
Philippines							
All	347	399	295	222	198	168	139
New S +	140	125	118	99	100	88	77
Viet Nam							
All	76	99	111	112	112	117	115
New S +	51	65	70	70	68	69	68
Western Pacific Region							
All	48	58	51	51	49	49	48
New S +	20	22	23	24	24	23	22

FIGURE 5

Trend in notification of smear-positive cases (rate per 100 000) in Cambodia, China, the Philippines and Viet Nam, Western Pacific Region, 1995–2001

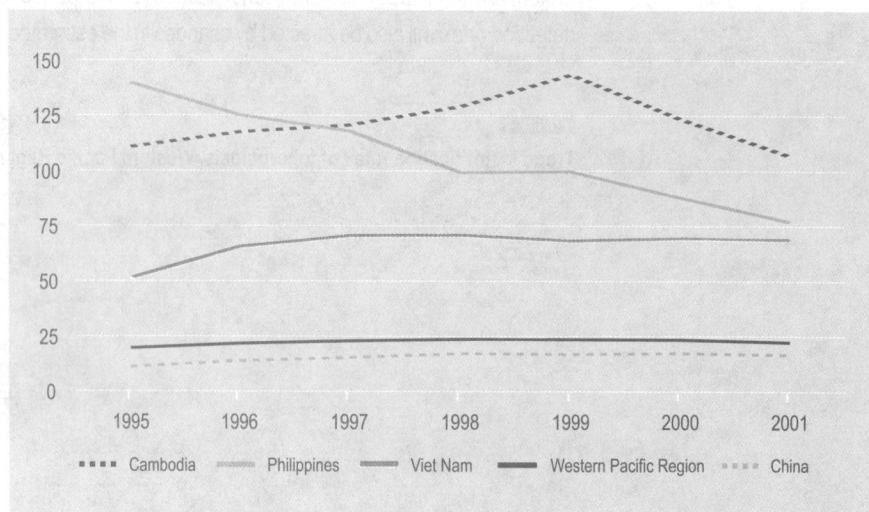

1.5 Prevalence of HIV infection among tuberculosis patients

Tuberculosis patients have been included in the surveillance sentinel groups for human immunodeficiency virus (HIV) infection prevalence surveys in Cambodia and Viet Nam. HIV sero-prevalence in newly detected tuberculosis cases increased from 6% in 2000 to 8.4% in Cambodia (2002 survey). HIV sero-prevalence in 2001 was 4.9% in Malaysia; 3% in Fiji; 1.2% in New Zealand; 1% in Papua New Guinea and the Northern Mariana Islands; 0.5% in Hong Kong, China and Macao, China; and 0.3% in Singapore.

1.6 Primary multidrug resistance

Primary multidrug resistance (combined resistance to at least rifampicin and isoniazide) was found in China in 2000, ranging from 2.9% to 5.3% of newly detected cases in three provinces (Guangdong 5.3%, Zhejiang 4.3% and Shandong 2.9%) (see profiles of high-burden countries in Annex 1).

CHAPTER 2

Review of DOTS implementation and treatment results

Twenty-two
countries
achieved 97%
DOTS coverage
or above.

Among the 33 countries and areas of the Region that reported in 2001, 30 had at least part of their population served by DOTS units, compared to 18 in 1998. Twenty-nine countries had a tuberculosis manual, 20 had a special budget for tuberculosis control, 26 had a centralized system for the procurement and distribution of tuberculosis drugs, 15 had a system to prevent the sale of rifampicin to the general public, 22 had a reference laboratory and 19 had a mechanism for collecting notification of tuberculosis cases from private practitioners.

2.1 Population with access to DOTS

The population in the Region with access to DOTS increased slightly from 67% in 2000 to 68% in 2001 (Table 1, page viii). DOTS was applied in 52% of operational health units (2528 out of 4841) in the Region; for China, the percentage was 49% (1560 out of 3164 health units).

Twenty-two countries achieved 97% DOTS coverage or above (American Samoa; Brunei Darussalam; Cambodia; Cook Islands; Fiji; French Polynesia; Guam; Hong Kong, China; Kiribati; Macao, China; Malaysia; the Marshall Islands; Mongolia; Nauru; New Zealand; Niue; the Northern Mariana Islands; the Philippines; Samoa; Singapore; Tonga; and Viet Nam). The population with access to DOTS was 90% in Solomon Islands, 80% in the Lao Peoples' Democratic Republic, 70% in the Federated States of Micronesia, 68% in China, 65% in Vanuatu, 54% in Australia, 46% in Japan and 13% in Papua New Guinea. Among the countries that made the biggest progress compared to the previous year were Vanuatu (50% to 65%), Japan (36% to 46%), the Lao People's Democratic Republic (70% to 80%), the Philippines (90% to 97%) and Papua New Guinea (8% to 13%) (Table 1).

2.2 DOTS enrolment

In 2001, 78% of all cases and 89% of new smear-positive cases in the Region were diagnosed and treated under DOTS (Table 1). This marks a rapid improvement since 1999, when the figures were 69% for all cases and 78% for new smear-positive cases. The increase was particularly marked in the Philippines (from 28% in 1999 to 100% in 2001) and Japan (from 37% in 1999 to 50% in 2001).

FIGURE 6

Trends in population with access to DOTS and DOTS enrolment rate (all cases) in the Western Pacific Region, 1998–2001

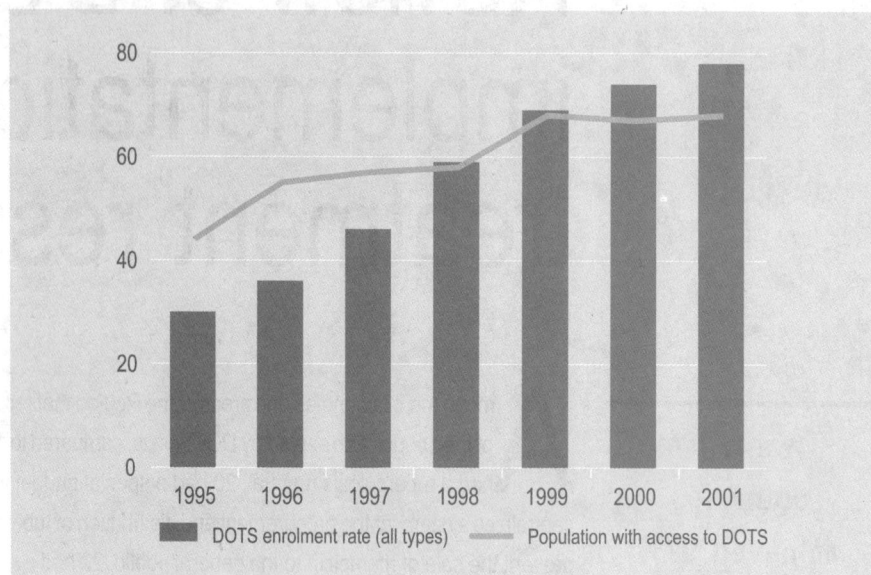

2.3 Treatment results of new smear-positive cases

In DOTS areas, the treatment success rate was 92.3% for the cohort of 320 046 new pulmonary smear-positive cases treated in 2000 (they represented 83% of the 385 434 cases notified that year) (Table 16, page 28). The cure rate among reported cases was 88.9%, completed treatment 3.5%, defaulted 2%, treatment failures 1.1%, died 1.9% and transferred out 1.4%. The percentage of cases not evaluated was 1.3%. In China, 89% of new smear-positive cases were registered for treatment results (191 280 out of 213 766 notified in 2000) and the treatment success rate was 95%.

In non-DOTS areas, the treatment success rate was 69.8% out of 38 139 cases (which in turn comprise 66% of the 57 741 cases notified in 2000) (Table 17, page 29). In China, 97% of the 22 486 cases notified in 2000 were evaluated and the treatment success was 81.3%.

> **In DOTS areas, the treatment success rate was 92.3% for the cohort of 320 046 new pulmonary smear-positive cases treated in 2000.**

2.4 Treatment results of re-treatment cases

In DOTS areas, 54 043 re-treatment cases registered in 2000 were evaluated (including relapses, failures and returns after treatment interruption). The treatment success rate for these was 86.6%. The cure rate was 83.5%, completed treatment 3%, defaulted 1.3%, treatment failures 2%, died 2.2%, transferred out 0.9% and 7.2% of the cases were not evaluated (Table 18, page 30).

In non-DOTS areas, the treatment success rate for re-treatment cases was 31.3% (Table 19, page 31). Out of 728 re-treated cases registered in 2000, 57% were not evaluated; therefore, the cure rate was only 23%, completed treatment 8.4%, defaulted 2.2%, treatment failures 4.1%, died 2.1% and transferred out 3.6%.

FIGURE 7

Treatment success in DOTS and non-DOTS areas, 2000 cohort

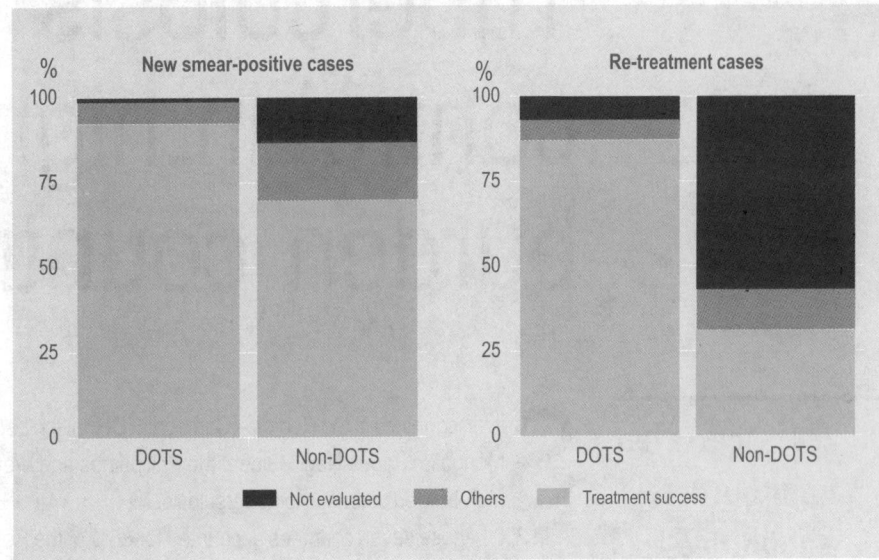

CHAPTER 3

Tuberculosis control in high-burden countries

In 2001, the seven high-burden countries accounted for 86% of the Region's population and 94% of all estimated incident cases (or more than 1.9 million new cases by year).

Seven countries in the Region – Cambodia, China, the Lao People's Democratic Republic, Mongolia, Papua New Guinea, the Philippines and Viet Nam – have been identified as high-burden countries for tuberculosis.

In 2001, these seven countries accounted for 86% of the Region's population and 94% of all estimated incident cases (or more than 1.9 million new cases by year). They notified 88% of all cases (711 581 out of 811 263 cases) and 91% of the smear-positive cases in the Region (344 296 out of 379 060 cases). The average case detection was 33% for all types and 40% for the new smear-positive cases. DOTS expansion made the best progress in this group of countries. In 2001, 71% of the population of these countries had access to DOTS and the DOTS enrolment rate for pulmonary new smear-positive cases was 83%. Treatment success exceeded 85% in five of these countries, including China. Mongolia and Viet Nam have reached the targets of 70% case detection and 85% treatment success (for new smear-positive cases). In 2001, Mongolia passed the WHO targets for the first time, two years after achieving full DOTS coverage in 1999. Viet Nam has been maintaining high case detection and treatment success for several years. Cambodia, China and the Philippines have all exceeded the 85% treatment success target.

3.1 Tuberculosis control policies and DOTS components in high-burden countries

All high-burden countries are using WHO-recommended national tuberculosis guidelines and have central procurement and distribution systems for tuberculosis drugs as well as a national reference laboratory. Five countries allot a separate budget for tuberculosis control. DOTS is implemented in all public hospitals in Cambodia, Mongolia, the Philippines and Viet Nam, and in 80% of hospitals in the Lao People's Democratic Republic, 58% in China and 13% in Papua New Guinea. Most of the countries use sputum smear microscopy for diagnosis, the exception being Papua New Guinea, where it is used in some units only. Directly observed treatment (DOT) is applied in all public health units within DOTS areas. Treatment and smear microscopy examinations are free of charge for the patients in six countries, while China has a patient fee system. Reporting of treatment results is based on cohort analysis in all units in Cambodia, the Lao People's Democratic Republic, Mongolia, Papua New Guinea and Viet Nam, and in some units in China and the Philippines. Screening and treatment of contact children is carried out in some units only.

3.2 Notification in high-burden countries

In 2001, the notification rate for all cases exceeded 100 per 100 000 population in four of the seven high-burden countries: 143 in Cambodia, 139 in the Philippines, 138 in Mongolia and 115 in Viet Nam. These seven notified a higher proportion of pulmonary smear-positive cases (48% of all cases) than other areas of the Region, where they accounted for 35% of all cases. The estimated incidence[4] of smear-positive cases was 59 per 100 000 in the seven high-burden countries, compared to 22 per 100 000 in the others. However, at 40%, the case detection rate for smear-positives was lower in the high-burden countries compared to 66% in the other countries. The case detection rate was 34% in China, where more than 70% of the estimated cases of the Region reside; therefore DOTS expansion in China is a pre-condition for reaching the WHO target of 70% case finding in the Region.

The notification rate of new smear-positive cases increased between the years 1995 and 2001 in Mongolia. It also rose slightly in China, the Lao People's Democratic Republic and Viet Nam. Cambodia and the Philippines have seen a decrease since 1999. Fluctuations in the Papua New Guinea results are mostly due to significant variations in the reporting system; only the cases registered in DOTS areas were reported in 2001 (Figure 8, below).

FIGURE 8

Trend in notification rate (per 100 000) of new smear-positive cases, high tuberculosis burden countries in the Western Pacific Region, 1995–2001

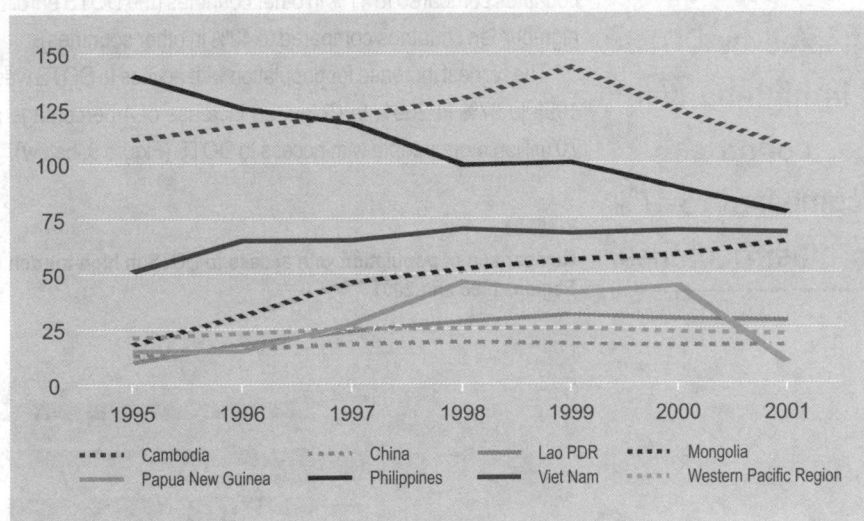

3.3 DOTS implementation in high-burden countries

DOTS has made faster progress in high-burden countries than in others. By the end of 2001, 71% of their population had access to DOTS, compared to 47% in other countries. Nearly all of the populations of Cambodia, Mongolia and Viet Nam can access DOTS. DOTS coverage has also risen to 97% in the Philippines (from 75% in 2000), 80% in the Lao People's Democratic Republic (from 70% in 2000), and 13% in Papua New Guinea (from 8% in 2000). The proportion of population with access to DOTS in China remained the same as the previous year at 68% (Table 3, overleaf).

---

[4] Based on the 2001 update of estimated cases from WHO, Geneva.

TABLE 3

DOTS in high-burden countries, Western Pacific Region, 1998–2001 (%)

	Population with access to DOTS		Case detection rate* new S+		DOTS enrolment new S+		DOTS case detection rate* new S+	
Country	1998	2001	1998*	2001**	1998	2001	1998	2001
Cambodia	100	100	54	41	100	100	54	41
China	64	68	33	33	89	89	30	29
Lao PDR	71	80	39	27	99	100	39	27
Mongolia	97	100	57	72	89	100	51	72
Papua New Guinea	9	13	41	9	20	100	8	9
Philippines	17	97	70	57	14	100	10	57
Viet Nam	96	100	83	84	97	100	81	84
High-burden countries	**63**	**71**	**43**	**40**	**76**	**93**	**32**	**37**
Other countries	24	47	66	66	33	47	22	31
Western Pacific Region	58	68	44	41	72	89	32	37

* Case detection rates and DOTS case detection rates have been made available since the publication of estimated cases in Global Burden of Tuberculosis, 1999.
** Updated estimates are given for 2001.

> **About 93% of the new pulmonary smear-positive cases were detected and treated by DOTS in high-burden countries compared to 47% in other countries.**

The DOTS enrolment rate is also much greater in the high-burden countries. About 93% of the new pulmonary smear-positive cases were detected and treated by DOTS in high-burden countries compared to 47% in other countries (the DOTS enrolment rate was 83% for all types in high-burden countries compared to 42% in other countries).

The highest increase for population with access to DOTS was in the Philippines – from 17% in 1998 to 97% in 2001. In China, an increase of 4 percentage points since 1998 translates as 70 million more people with access to DOTS (Figure 9, below).

FIGURE 9

Comparison of population with access to DOTS in high-burden countries, Western Pacific Region, 1998 and 2001

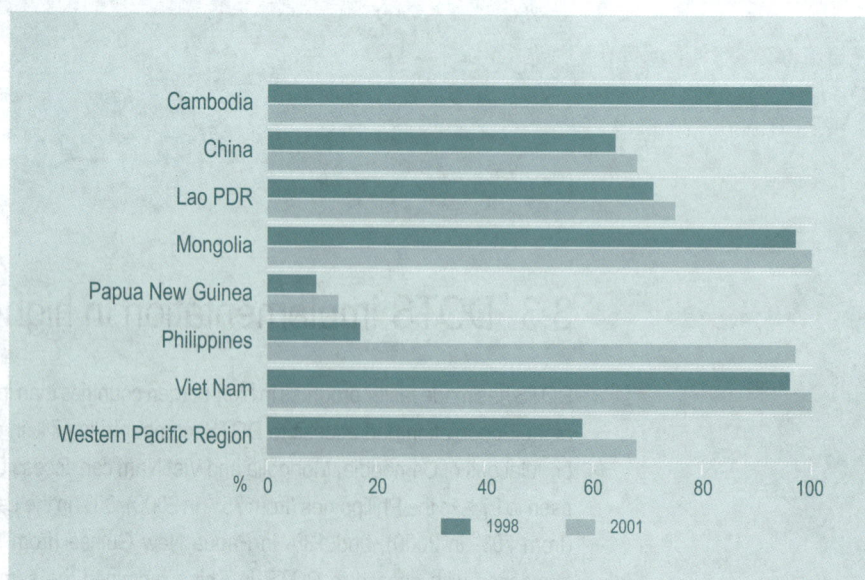

3.4 Treatment results in high-burden countries

Better treatment outcomes were observed in the high-burden countries with the greatest DOTS enrolment. Treatment success in DOTS areas was 93% in high-burden countries (new smear-positive cases registered in 2000), compared to 73% in other countries. The proportion of patients not evaluated[5] was only 1% in high-burden countries, compared to 9% in other countries (Table 4, below).

The cure rate was 90% in high-burden countries (53% in others), died 1.7% (8.3% in others), treatment failure 1% (5.4%) and defaulted 2% (2.7%) (Table 4). Patients treated under DOTS benefited from better management and follow-up (including sputum examinations at the end of treatment to confirm that the patient had been "cured").

By country, the treatment success for pulmonary new smear-positive cases exceeded 85% in five countries, while it was 82% in the Lao People's Democratic Republic (compared to 62% in 1997) and 63% in Papua New Guinea (Table 4). The Philippines' figures improved from 83% in 1997 to 88% in 2001. Cambodia, China and Viet Nam have also maintained high treatment success rates since 1997.

TABLE 4

Treatment outcomes of new smear-positive cases in seven high-burden countries, cohort 2000 in DOTS areas, Western Pacific Region

Country	Registered number	Not evaluated (%)	Cured (%)	Completed treatment (%)	Defaulted (%)	Failed (%)	Died (%)	Transferred out (%)	Treatment success (%)*
Cambodia	14 775	0.0	87.8	3.5	3.9	0.3	3.6	0.8	91.4
China	19 1280	1.8	94.6	0.0	0.8	1.0	1.0	0.9	94.6
Lao PDR	1392	0.0	72.8	8.7	8.5	0.4	6.8	2.8	81.5
Mongolia	1389	0.1	83.2	3.7	4.2	3.3	2.7	2.8	86.8
Papua New Guinea	422	4.7	38.6	24.2	25.6	0.5	2.4	4.0	62.8
Philippines	50 196	0.1	72.6	15.2	5.8	1.2	2.3	2.8	87.8
Viet Nam	53 169	0.1	89.9	2.2	1.8	1.0	3.1	1.9	92.1
High-burden countries	312 623	1.1	89.7	3.1	2.0	1.0	1.7	1.4	92.8
Other countries	7396	8.8	52.6	20.2	2.7	5.4	8.3	2.1	72.8
Western Pacific Region	320 019	1.3	88.9	3.5	2.0	1.1	1.9	1.4	92.3

*Treatment success is the sum of cured and completed treatment.

---

[5] Among the cohort of new smear-positive pulmonary patients registered for a treatment outcome in 2000.

PART II
Tables

Table 5
Notification of tuberculosis cases by type, Western Pacific Region, 2001   17

Table 6
Age and sex distribution of new sputum smear-positive cases in DOTS and
non-DOTS areas, Western Pacific Region, 2001   18

Table 7
Notification rate per 100 000 of new smear-positive cases by age and sex in
DOTS and non-DOTS areas,Western Pacific Region, 2001   19

Table 8
Trend in notified tuberculosis cases (all types) in DOTS and non-DOTS areas   20

Table 9
Trend in notified cases (new smear-positives) in DOTS and non-DOTS areas   21

Table 10
Trend in tuberculosis notification rates per 100 000 population (all types)   22

Table 11
Trend in tuberculosis notification rates per 100 000 population (smear-positives)   23

Table 12
Trend in tuberculosis notification (number of all types) in DOTS and
non-DOTS areas, 1998–2001   24

Table 13
Trend in tuberculosis notification (number of new smear-positives) in DOTS and
non-DOTS areas, 1998–2001   24

Table 14
Trend in tuberculosis notification (rate for all types) in DOTS and non-DOTS areas, 1998–2001   26

Table 15
Trend in tuberculosis notification (rate for new smear-positives) in DOTS and
non-DOTS areas, 1998–2001   26

Table 16
Treatment outcome of new smear-positive cases registered in 2000 in DOTS areas   28

Table 17
Treatment outcome of new smear-positive cases registered in 2000 in non-DOTS areas   29

Table 18
Treatment outcome of re-treatment cases registered in 2000 in DOTS areas   30

Table 19
Treatment outcome of re-treatment cases registered in 2000 in non-DOTS areas   31

Tables

TABLE 5

Notification of tuberculosis cases by type, Western Pacific Region, 2001

Country	Pulmonary — Sputum positive: New	% out of the total	% out of new pulmonary	Relapse	% of all S+ out of all pulmonary	Sputum negative	% out of the total	Extra-pulmonary	% out of the total	All types
American Samoa	2	67	100	0	100	0	0	1	33	3
Australia	228	23	46	29	52	236	24	372	38	980
Brunei Darussalam	95		53	9	58	74	34	27	13	216
Cambodia	14 361	75	86	721	90	1658	9	2430	13	19 170
China	212 766	44	49	19 729	53	203 252	42	0		485 221
Cook Islands	2	100	100	0	100	0	0	0	0	2
Fiji	73	40	54	1	54	62	34	47	26	183
French Polynesia	24	53	80	0	80	6	13	8	18	45
Guam	47	75	94	1	96	2	3	3	5	63
Hong Kong, China	1853	26	34	233	39	3294	45	824	11	7262
Japan	11 408	32	41	1248	46	14 836	42	6621	19	35 489
Kiribati	64	34	68	6	74	24	13	74	39	189
Republic of Korea	11 805	32	40	3145	50	14 912	40	3797	10	37 268
Lao PDR	1533	64	71	85	75	533	22	231	10	2382
Macao, China	157	34	40	26	47	206	44	48	10	465
Malaysia	8309	56	62	0	62	5139	35	1382	9	14 830
N. Mariana Islands	19	33	38	0	38	31	53	8		58
Marshall Islands	15	27	39	0	39	23	41	14	25	56
Micronesia, FS	8	8	26	0	26	23	24	21	22	95
Mongolia	1631	46	65	113	70	757	21	1025	29	3526
Nauru	2	67	67	0	67	1	33	0	0	3
New Caledonia	34	53	68	2	72	14	22	14	22	64
New Zealand	68	18	48	11	56	63	17	108	29	377
Niue	0			0		0		0		0
Palau										0
Papua New Guinea	462	13	23	29	25	1496	43	1483	43	3470
Philippines	59 341	55	55	5379	60	42 413	40	0	0	107 133
Pitcairn Islands										0
Samoa	12	55	75	1	81	3	14	6	27	22
Singapore	357	23	28	62	33	861	56	196	13	1536
Solomon Islands	118	40	50	0	50	118	40	54	18	292
Tokelau	0			0		0		0		0
Tonga	8	73	80	1	90	1	9	1	9	11
Tuvalu										0
Vanuatu	56	32	40	0	40	84	49	33	19	173
Viet Nam	54 202	60	71	5347	78	17 106	19	14 024	15	90 679
Wallis and Futuna										0
Total	**379 060**	**47**	**52**	**36 178**	**57**	**307 228**	**38**	**32 852**	**4**	**811 263**

TABLE 6

Age and sex distribution of new sputum smear-positive (S+) cases in DOTS and non-DOTS areas, Western Pacific Region,* 2001

Country	New S+ males								New S+ females								New S+ males and females							
	0-14	15-24	25-34	35-44	45-54	55-64	>=65	Total	0-14	15-24	25-34	35-44	45-54	55-64	>=65	Total	0-14	15-24	25-34	35-44	45-54	55-64	>=65	Total
American Samoa	0	0	0	0	0	0	0	0	0	0	0	1	0	1	0	2	0	0	0	1	0	1	0	2
Australia	1	23	20	18	18	13	35	128	1	21	27	16	7	8	20	100	2	44	47	34	25	21	55	228
Brunei Darussalam	0	0	0	0	0	0	0	0	0	0	0	0	0	0	0	0	0	0	0	0	0	0	0	0
Cambodia	29	600	1302	1601	1406	1403	1037	7378	25	455	1033	1526	1687	1428	829	6983	54	1055	2335	3127	3093	2831	1866	14 361
China	1213	19 121	28 520	25 544	25 759	20 789	22 799	143 745	1405	14 500	17 446	12 041	9963	7175	6491	69 021	2618	33 621	45 966	37 585	35 722	27 964	29 290	212 766
Cook Islands	0	0	0	0	0	0	2	2	0	0	0	0	0	0	0	0	0	0	0	0	0	0	2	2
Fiji	0	6	8	11	7	4	2	38	0	7	5	7	1	2	2	24	0	13	13	18	8	6	4	62
French Polynesia	2	5	1	2	4	4	5	23	3	7	1	3	3	4	1	22	5	12	7	3	13	8	7	45
Guam	0	1	4	10	9	3	6	33	0	2	3	3	4	2	1	15	0	3	7	13	13	5	7	48
Hong Kong, China	6	79	100	162	196	200	518	1261	13	88	119	83	58	34	197	592	19	167	219	245	254	234	715	1853
Japan	3	220	576	632	1319	1513	3840	8103	5	175	437	228	250	330	1880	3305	8	395	1013	860	1569	1843	5720	11 408
Kiribati	4	10	7	3	5	5	1	35	4	7	7	3	3	4	1	29	8	17	14	6	8	9	4	64
Republic of Korea	23	942	1415	1419	1293	1103	1361	7556	45	839	890	489	326	390	1270	4249	68	1781	2305	1908	1619	1493	2631	11 805
Lao PDR	8	79	136	172	215	182	161	953	6	51	97	119	134	102	66	575	14	130	233	291	349	284	227	1528
Macao, China	0	9	17	26	25	11	23	111	1	5	7	11	10	1	11	46	1	14	24	37	35	12	34	157
Malaysia	48	713	1198	1221	1011	934	738	5863	36	510	506	445	374	353	222	2446	84	1223	1704	1666	1385	1287	960	8309
N. Mariana Islands	0	1	3	0	2	2	2	10	0	5	4	0	2	2	1	9	0	6	7	0	4	2	0	19
Marshall Islands	3	8	4	2	4	2	0	23	5	6	4	7	8	2	1	33	8	14	8	9	12	4	1	56
Micronesia, FS	0	2	0	0	2	1	0	5	1	0	1	0	0	1	0	3	1	2	1	0	2	2	0	8
Mongolia	13	236	268	179	86	45	36	863	25	253	260	125	48	28	29	768	38	489	528	304	134	73	65	1631
Nauru	0	0	1	1	0	0	0	2	0	1	0	0	0	0	0	1	0	1	1	1	0	0	0	3
New Caledonia	0	1	7	1	5	6	6	26	1	2	0	1	0	0	3	8	1	2	9	2	5	6	9	34
New Zealand	1	7	2	7	4	2	12	35	3	9	14	3	1	3	5	38	4	16	16	10	5	5	17	73
Niue	0	0	0	0	0	0	0	0	0	0	0	0	0	0	0	0	0	0	0	0	0	0	0	0
Palau	0	0	0	0	0	0	0	0	0	0	0	0	0	0	0	0	0	0	0	0	0	0	0	0
Papua New Guinea	4	101	72	29	26	9	4	245	7	91	64	32	17	5	1	217	11	192	136	61	43	14	5	462
Philippines	0	0	0	0	0	0	0	0	0	0	0	0	0	0	0	0	0	0	0	0	0	0	0	0
Pitcairn Islands	0	0	0	0	0	0	0	0	0	0	0	0	0	0	0	0	0	0	0	0	0	0	0	0
Samoa	1	3	1	1	0	0	1	7	0	1	1	2	1	1	1	7	1	4	2	3	1	1	2	14
Singapore	1	6	19	39	70	66	76	277	1	5	7	19	15	9	24	80	2	11	26	58	85	75	100	357
Solomon Islands	31	25	24	20	19	21	8	148	31	31	29	15	24	7	3	140	62	56	53	35	43	28	11	288
Tokelau	0	0	0	0	0	0	0	0	0	0	0	0	0	0	0	0	0	0	0	0	0	0	0	0
Tonga	0	0	1	0	0	2	1	4	0	0	2	1	1	0	0	4	0	0	3	1	1	2	1	8
Tuvalu	0	0	0	0	0	0	0	0	0	0	0	0	0	0	0	0	0	0	0	0	0	0	0	0
Vanuatu	0	8	5	4	8	4	0	29	1	9	4	4	3	5	0	26	1	17	9	8	11	9	0	55
Viet Nam	39	2756	6319	8457	7054	5205	7643	37 473	48	1390	2357	2656	2574	2530	5174	16 729	87	4146	8676	11 113	9628	7735	12 817	54 202
Wallis and Futuna	0	0	0	0	0	0	0	0	0	0	0	0	0	0	0	0	0	0	0	0	0	0	0	0
Western Pacific Region	1430	24 962	40 030	39 561	38 547	31 529	38 317	214 376	1667	18 468	23 327	17 838	15 513	12 425	16 234	105 472	3097	43 430	63 357	57 399	54 060	43 954	54 551	319 848
%	1	12	19	18	18	15	18	100.00	2	18	22	17	15	12	15	100.00	1	14	20	18	17	14	17	100.00

*Breakdown of cases by age and sex was not available for the Philippines.

TABLE 7

Notification rate per 100 000 of new sputum smear-positive cases by age and sex in DOTS and non-DOTS areas, Western Pacific Region, 2001

	Western Pacific Region*	Population	Number of new S+ cases	Rates per 100 000
Males	0–14	208 696 710	1430	0.7
	15–24	130 963 661	24 962	19.1
	25–34	154 190 079	40 030	26.0
	35–44	120 294 576	39 561	32.9
	45–54	95 722 295	38 547	40.3
	55–64	59 709 423	31 529	52.8
	>=65	54 667 272	38 317	70.1
	Total	**824 244 016**	**214 376**	**26.0**
Females	0–14	189 488 306	1667	0.9
	15–24	122 365 550	18 468	15.1
	25–34	147 455 225	23 327	15.8
	35–44	114 644 560	17 838	15.6
	45–54	91 278 229	15 513	17.0
	55–64	57 526 734	12 425	21.6
	>=65	67 348 448	16 234	24.1
	Total	**790 107 052**	**105 472**	**13.3**
Males and females	0–14	398 185 016	3097	0.8
	15–24	253 329 211	43 430	17.1
	25–34	301 645 304	63 357	21.0
	35–44	234 939 136	57 399	24.4
	45–54	187 000 524	54 060	28.9
	55–64	117 236 157	43 954	37.5
	>=65	122 015 720	54 551	44.7
	Total	**1 614 351 068**	**319 848**	**19.8**

Trend in notified tuberculosis cases (all types) in DOTS and non-DOTS areas

Year	WPR	Wallis and Futuna	Viet Nam	Vanuatu	Tuvalu	Tonga	Tokelau	Solomon Islands	Singapore	Samoa	Pitcairn Islands	Philippines	Papua New Guinea	Palau	Niue	New Zealand	New Caledonia	Nauru	Mongolia	Micronesia, FS	Marshall Islands	N. Mariana Islands	Malaysia	Macao, China	Lao PDR	Republic of Korea	Kiribati	Japan	Hong Kong, China	Guam	French Polynesia	Fiji	Cook Islands	China	Cambodia	Brunei Darussalam	Australia	American Samoa
1977	222 855			150		62		355	2760	36		107 108	2212	7		608			1075								97	89 245	7191	67	95	257					1251	7
1978	294 647		68 650	131		89		411	2964	59		118 587	2446	14		595			1107		8						40	80 629	6623	64	78	183	30			230	1292	8
1979	308 161		11 821	184	7	71		452	2800	58		108 813	2232	9		542			1123		6			442		81 910	94	76 455	7903	71	81	205	37			216	1542	2
1980	346 198		43 062	178	33	64		266	2710	59		112 307	2525	17		474	108		1160		4		11 168	1101		89 803	146	70 916	8065	55	73	210	10			196	1457	2
1981	353 240		43 506	92	18	49		313	2425	49		116 821	2418	10		448	128		1094	67	6	26	10 970	585		98 532	187	65 867	7729	41	58	180	19			285	1386	6
1982	355 645		51 206	173	12	45		324	2179	43		104 715	2742	17		437	107		1325	73	7	75	11 894	455		91 572	193	63 940	7527	49	48	163	29	98 654	8158	245	1270	6
1983	457 427		43 185	171	23	50	0	302	2065	41		106 300	2954	14		415	161		1514	75	12	74	11 634	671		85 669	127	62 021	7301	48	66	185	20	117 557	7572	276	1219	8
1984	534 450		43 875	188	9	54	0	337	2143	37		151 863	3505	20		402	144		1652	66	15	58	10 577	571		87 169	111	61 521	7843	54	73	165	36	151 564	7906	256	1299	12
1985	611 088		46 941	124	32	49	2	377	1952			151 028	3678	26		359	104		2994	60	12	64	10 569			88 789	103	58 567	7545	37	75	230	17	226 899	10 145	238	1088	5
1986	650 256		47 557	131	27	35		292	1760	29		153 129	2877	13		320	98		2819	97	37	16	10 735	420		87 419	129	56 690	7432	49	79	199	16	265 095	10 325	212	906	8
1987	714 475		55 505	90	22	24	9	334	1616	29		163 740	3235	38		296	74		2433	77	32	49	11 068	389		74 460	110	56 496	7269	34	63	173	15	313 604	9106	189	907	9
1988	766 627		52 463	118	24	14	1	372	1666	37		183 113	4261	17		295	111		2538	68	11	27	10 944	320		70 012	208	54 357	7021	41	64	162	1	362 114	10 691	126	954	13
1989	796 087		52 270	144	25	35		488	1617			217 272	3396	3	2	303	110		2233		7	28	10 686	274			121	53 112	6704	75	58	218	1	367 799	7906	128	952	5
1990	888 409		47 536	140	23	23	1	382	1591	44		317 008	2497	6	1	348	130		1659				10 873	343		63 904	68	51 821	6510	40	59	252	1	375 481	6501	143	1016	15
1991	784 409		54 509	234	16	19		309	1512	26		207 371	3401		2	335	140		1611	111	52	67	11 059	329	1951	57 864		50 612	6283	49	49	210	12	376 246	10 903	160	950	2
1992	433 480	4	56 594	147	30	23		364	1722	49	0	236 172	2540	25	1	317	140		1516	151	61	46	11 420	294	994	48 070	100	48 956	6534	70	83	240	6	344 218	16 148	0	1011	
1993	711 162		52 994	114	28	32		367	1677	45	0	174 189	5516	41	2	274	149	4	1418	171	0	40	12 075	318	1905	46 999	253	47 437	6537	94	82	166	4	363 804	13 270	0	991	4
1994	723 716	11	51 763	152	19	23	1	332	1889	51	0	180 044	5335	19	1	352	132	0	1730	0	49	66	11 708	349	1135	44 590	0	44 016	6319	0	89	225	1	357 829	15 112	0	1073	
1995	774 721	4	55 739	79	36	20		352	1889	37	0	235 496	8041	5	2	307	0	0	3010	94	42	75	11 778	354	1307	43 078	327	43 078	6212	0	0	203	2	469 358	14 599	0	1073	6
1996	942 481	0	74 711	0	0	22	1	289	1977	32	0	276 295	5087	15	1	323	205	0	3010	108	34	0	12 902	455	1440	42 122	32	42 122	6501	75	86	200	3	418 903	14 857	0	1073	0
1997	834 722	14	84 964	184	0	21	0	318	2120	22	0	208 301	7977	0	2	328	0	0	2987	138	91	93	13 539	589	1923	42 190	276	42 190	6983	70	91	171	0	457 349	15 629	0	1145	6
1998	839 121	0	87 449	178	18	30	1	295	1654	31	0	159 866	11 291	32	1	367	102	0	2915	102	42	97	14 115	463	2165	44 016	253	44 016	7673	94	105	166	2	460 169	16 946	272	899	0
1999	823 421	0	88 879	117	0	22	0	289	1728	43	0	145 807	12 189	0	2	348	86	4	3348	91	34	66	14 908	0	2437	40 800	210	40 800	7087	54	93	192	3	463 373	19 266	307	1073	4
2000	806 970	0	89 792	152	0	24	0	303	1728	43	0	128 495	12 121	0	1	344	86	0	3109	91	56	75	15 057	449	2234	21 782	210	39 384	7578	54	59	144	1	463 373	18 891	307	1043	3
2001	811 263	0	90 679	173	0	11	0	292	1536	22	0	107 133	3470	0	0	377	64	3	3526	95	56	58	14 830	465	2382	37 268	189	35 489	7262	63	45	183	2	485 221	19 170	216	980	3

20

TABLE 9

Trend in notified tuberculosis cases (new smear-positives) in DOTS and non-DOTS areas

	1977	1978	1979	1980	1981	1982	1983	1984	1985	1986	1987	1988	1989	1990	1991	1992	1993	1994	1995	1996	1997	1998	1999	2000	2001
WPR	22 917	22 934	57 388	78 049	118 202	148 558	150 982	161 230	208 493	226 410	186 522	178 366	199 654	94 522	100 286	184 312	267 476	282 061	314 624	352 935	375 801	393 244	393 801	385 434	379 060
Wallis and Futuna																	2	0		0	1	0	0	0	0
Viet Nam					33 243	33 014	32 612	30 426	34 217	30 381	34 530	39 486	35 095	30 728	35 865	38 659	36 534	35 613	37 550	48 911	53 647	54 873	53 805	53 169	54 202
Vanuatu	57	52	52	59	34	49	55	55	51	36	26	46	39			84	41	62	30	0	66	38	43	63	56
Tuvalu				23	10	3	7	3	3	5	7	7	2	7	5	5	2	1	6	0	0	0	0	0	0
Tonga	29	41	28	32	18	25	23	25	23	18	12	7	16		17	17	16	17	9	16	12	16	10	15	8
Tokelau																	0	0	0	1	0	0	0	0	0
Solomon Islands	182	174	184	153	174	176	130	155	155	101	115	137	149	117	88	130	155	114	109	90	113	140	93	109	118
Singapore	1285	1375	1197	1266	1062	998	860	992	949	839	740	794	823	840		841		861	455	455	432	480	465	248	357
Samoa					32	30	25	20								2	21	18	15	10	14	7	17	13	12
Pitcairn Islands																				0	0	0	0	0	0
Philippines				17 275	19 006	20 676	18 657	21 291	39 571	50 624	72 150	63 655	97 070			92 279	87 401	94 768	86 695	83 353	71 663	73 373	67 056	59 341	
Papua New Guinea	852	903	883	967	867	942	870	1061	870	606	839	1273	951	611	489		812	573	1652	652	1195	2107	1914	2267	462
Palau				10	5	2	6		4	0	4					8	11	9	4	7	0	20	0	0	
Niue																	0	0	1	1	0	0	1	0	0
New Zealand									69	66	55		62				91	61	47	76	57	81	69	74	68
New Caledonia						34	60						40	37	33	32	35	42	0	26	0	30	0	38	34
Nauru																2	0	0	0	0	0	0		4	2
Mongolia									363	320	271	276	234	185	128	92	87	200	622	622	1171	1356	1513	1389	1631
Micronesia, FS						11	32	18	14	10	18					19	8	15	0	10	11	28	16	15	8
Marshall Islands					5	4	6	6	7	8	4					14	12	0	17	0	11	17	15		
N. Mariana Islands				0	11	3	28	4	5	22					21		22	14	0	14	26	15	27	19	
Malaysia	6050	6313	6622	6819	6766	7320	7251	6660	6682	6653	6924	6718	6711	6774	6752	6754	6954	6861	6688	7271	7596	7802	7960	8156	8309
Macao, China												133		124	140	158	108	171	141	204	304	226	0	133	157
Lao PDR															526	459	765	752	726	886	1234	1508	1719	1526	1533
Republic of Korea			34 633	38 211	43 868	46 735	45 688	42 561	48 515	49 083	45 066	39 040	33 968	30 700	28 790	17 736	16 630	18 375	11 754	11 420	9957	10 359	9559	8 216	11 805
Kiribati	22	4	21	10	34	17	14										99	184	0	144	11	50	59	54	64
Japan	13 373	13 198	12 806	12 291	12 214	12 649	13 010	13 277	13 808	13 745	14 405	14 592	14 710	15 498	15 285	15 540	15 210	14 777	14 367	12 867	13 571	11 935	12 909	11 853	11 408
Hong Kong, China								4142	4110	4042	3918	3768	3670	3564		2429			0	2116	1536	1869	1566	1940	1853
Guam				53	40																		0	42	47
French Polynesia	41	32	41	52	39	32	48	52	48	49	45	44	43	34	40	39	38	0	37	41	34	33	29	24	
Fiji	145	101	114	111	97	98	79	82	99	86	75	65	76	83	63	75		60	68	69	66	74	65	62	73
Cook Islands										4	4	1	0			0		1	0	0	1	0	0	0	2
China					19 236	25 628	38 367	53 078	60 949							90 184	84 898	104 729	134 488	168 270	188 529	214 462	212 426	213 766	212 766
Cambodia			5801	5316	5507	5235	8715	7173	8246	5842	5132	8507		12 910	9560	11 058	11 101	12 065	12 686	13 865	15 744	14 822	14 361		
Brunei Darussalam			68	0	0			102	84																95
Australia	881	741	807	765	723	690	596	634	583						536	557		0		0	171	203	285	251	228
American Samoa				0	6	3	6	9	2	5	3						1		3	0	6	0	3	2	2

TABLE 10

Trend in tuberculosis notification rates per 100 000 population (all types)

Country	1976	1977	1978	1979	1980	1981	1982	1983	1984	1985	1986	1987	1988	1989	1990	1991	1992	1993	1994	1995	1996	1997	1998	1999	2000	2001
American Samoa	40	23	26	6	6	18	17	24	34	14	22	24	35	14	32	4		8		11	0	10	0	6	5	4
Australia	10	9	9	11	10	9	8	8	8	7	6	6	6	6	6	6	6	6		6	6	6	5	6	5	5
Brunei Darussalam	207		133	121	106	148	123	110	95	106	94	80	52		56		56	0	0	0			85	91		65
Cambodia			118	107	142	137	136	117	135	99	79	130	188	143		152	146	145	149	158	175	157				143
China			10	11	14	21	25	30	33	33	33	33	29	30	29		38	34	36	36	37					38
Cook Islands			167	206	59	106	161	105	180	85	94	88	5	6		71	32	21	5	0	0	10	15	6		10
Fiji	44	43	30	33	33	28	25	28	24	32	28	23	22	29	34	28	32		29	26	25	21	20	23	17	22
French Polynesia	81	68	55	55	49	39	31	40	46	47	44	37	34	32	33	27	45	39	41	0	39	40	46	40	26	19
Guam	58	82	76	68	51	37	49	42	45	31	40	27	33	60	32		49	64	0		0	0	0	35		40
Hong Kong, China	176	156	141	161	158	149	145	138	145	137	135	130	123	116	112	106	111	113	109	96	99	106	115	105	112	104
Japan	87	78	70	66	61	56	54	52	51	49	47	46	45	43	42	41	39	38	36	34	34	34	35	32	31	28
Kiribati	505	173	71	162	243	307	322	208	179	163	202	169	315	178	100		141		329	0	409	40	333	298	250	225
Republic of Korea			218	236	254		229	211	212	212	208	177	165	149		134	110	107	105	74	69	57	65	51	46	79
Lao PDR																45	23	41	24	27	29	37	40	44	42	44
Macao, China					411	196		150	217	146	101	94	72	60	76	70	77	83	88	80	103	134	105	0	103	104
Malaysia	89	80	80	83	81	78	82	78	70	67	67	66	65	62	61	60	61	63	59	58	63	64	66	68	68	66
N. Mariana Islands					153	441	435	305	320	80	136	71	74		146	98	66	0	143	139	89	109	76			
Marshall Islands	65	30	21	14	19	22	38	45	34	54	128	107	26	18		106	120		0	98	0	80	67	56	108	
Micronesia, FS						93	100	85	73	64	103	79	72		103	151	171	0	75	83	103	74	79	75		
Mongolia	76	71	71	70	71	65	77	86	91	162	148	125	127	109	79	75	69	64	77	122	120	116	111	125	131	138
Nauru																36	0	0	0	0	0	0	0	33		24
New Caledonia					78	90	72	111	95	69	66	48	69	69	79	84	82	85	74	0	111	0	50	0	41	29
New Zealand	20	20	19	17	15	14	14	13	12	11	10	9	9	9	10	10	9	8	10	9	5	9	10	9	9	10
Niue												67	50	100	50	100		50		100	50	0	50	100	0	0
Palau	38	50		100	64	113	67	142	100	154	217	93	271	121	25		50		156	256	112	29	88	0	178	0
Papua New Guinea	65	79	84	77	84	78	83	84	106	108	85	90	118	87	67	90	65	135	130	187	116	177	245	259	236	71
Philippines	338	238	260	234	233	236	204	204	284	276	274	279	308	362	516	330	377	269	272	347	399	295	222	198	168	139
Pitcairn Islands																										
Samoa	52	23	38	37	37	31	27	25	23		18	18	22		27		16	29	27	31	22	19	13	18	25	14
Singapore	123	119	126	117	112	99	88	83	84	76	68	62	63	60	59		54	62	59	57	56	57	61	47	53	37
Solomon Islands	154	172	192	205	118	134	130	117	125	140	102	116	122	153	120	94	109	104	91	93	74	79	71	63	74	63
Tokelau							0			0	100		450	50		50		50		0	50	50	0	0	0	0
Tonga	74	68	95	75	69	52	45	48	56	49	36	25	15	29	23	19	23	33	23	20	22	21	30	22	24	11
Tuvalu				100	471	225	150	288	113	400	338	275	300	313	288	200	375	311	211	360	0	0	180	0	0	0
Vanuatu	221	152	128	163	155	77	140	134	145	95	97	62	79	90	96	156	96	73	92	47	0	103	98	63	76	86
Viet Nam	115		134	23	80	79	91	76	75	78	77	86	82	81	72	81	82	74	71	76	999	111	112	112	117	115
Wallis and Futuna																	29		79	27	0	100	0	0	0	0
WPR																		45.7	45.5	48.2	57.9	50.8	50.6	49.2	49.0	47.7

TABLE 11

Trend in tuberculosis notification rates per 100 000 population (smear-positives)

Year	1976	1977	1978	1979	1980	1981	1982	1983	1984	1985	1986	1987	1988	1989	1990	1991	1992	1993	1994	1995	1996	1997	1998	1999	2000	2001
WPR																		16.6	17.5	19.6	21.7	22.9	23.7	23.5	23.4	22.3
Wallis and Futuna																			14	0	0	7	0	0	0	0
Viet Nam						61	59	57	52	57	49	53	62	54	47	53		56	51	49	51	65	70	70	68	68
Vanuatu	69	58	51	46	51	28	40	43	42	39	27	18	31	24		55	26	38	18	0	37	21	23	32		28
Tuvalu				329	125	38	88	38	38	63	88	88	25	88		63	63	22	11	60	0	0	0	0	0	0
Tonga	24	32	44	29	34	19	25	22	26	23	19	13	7		16	17	17	16	17	9	16	12	16	10	15	8
Tokelau															0			0	50	50	0	0	0			0
Solomon Islands	94	88	81	83	68	75	70	50	58	57	35	40	45	47	37	27	39	44	31	29	23	28	34	20	27	25
Singapore	59	55	58	50	52	43	40	34	39	37	32	28	30	31	31		30		31	14	13	13	14	13	8	9
Samoa						21	19	16	12							1	13	11	9	6	8	4	10	8	8	8
Pitcairn Islands																										
Philippines					36	38	40	36	40	72	90	123	107	162				142	132	140	125	118	99	100	88	77
Papua New Guinea		30	31	30	32	28	29	25	32	26	18	23	35	24	17	13		20	14	38	15	27	46	41	44	9
Palau						67	33	17	43		33	0	29					50	69	53	24	41	0	111	0	0
Niue																0		50	50	0	0	0	50	0		0
New Zealand										2	2	2	2			3	2	1	1		2	2	2	2		2
New Caledonia							23	41					25	23		20	19	20	24	0	14	0	15	0	18	15
Nauru														18				0	0		0		0		33	16
Mongolia										20	17	14	14	11	9	6	4	4	9	25	25	46	52	56	58	64
Micronesia, FS							15	44	20	15	11	19				18	8	15	0	8	8	21	12	13		6
Marshall Islands					16	13	19	18	20	29	14					29	24	0	30	0	18	27	18			29
N. Mariana Islands					0	65	18	147	20	25	61					46		47	23	0	22	37	20	39		25
Malaysia	53	47	48	49	50	48	50	49	44	42	41	41	40	39	38	37	36	37	35	33	35	36	36	36	37	37
Macao, China									29	27	30	41	28	43	32	46	69	51	51	30	30	35				35
Lao PDR																12	10	17	16	15	18	24	28	31	29	28
Republic of Korea				92	100	113	119	114	105	118	117	107	93	80	72	67	41	38	41	26	25	22	22	21	17	25
Kiribati	42	39	7	36	17	56	28	23								129	239	0	180	14	60	69	64			76
Japan	12	12	11	11	11	10	11	11	11	11	11	12	12	12	13	12	12	12	12	11	10	11	9	10	9	9
Hong Kong, China									75	75	72	69	65	63	60	42		0	32	23	0	28	23	29		27
Guam																37	27	0	0	0	0				27	30
French Polynesia	31	30	23	28	35	26	21	29	33	30	27	26	23	24		19	22	19	18	0	17	18	15	14	13	10
Fiji	21	24	17	18	18	15	15	12	12	14	12	10	9	10	11	8	10	8	9	9	8	9	8	7		9
Cook Islands										24	21	5	0	0	0	5		0								10
China						2	3	4	5	6						8	7	9	11	14	15	17	17	17	17	17
Cambodia						84	75	76	71	115	92	104	73	63		101	150	103	111	111	117	121	129	143	123	107
Brunei Darussalam																24		0	0		0		0	32	25	28
Australia	7	6	5	6	5	5	5	4	4	4						3	3	3	0	0	0	1	1	2	1	1
American Samoa					0	18	9	18	26	6	14	8				2		6			0	10	0	5	4	3

TABLE 12

Trend in tuberculosis notification (number of all types) in DOTS and non-DOTS areas, 1998–2001

Year		American Samoa	Australia	Brunei Darussalam	Cambodia	China	Cook Islands	Fiji	French Polynesia	Guam	Hong Kong, China	Japan	Kiribati	Republic of Korea	Lao PDR	Macao, China	Malaysia	N. Mariana Islands
1998	DOTS	6	424	0	16 946	336 535	2	166	105	0	0	0	276	30 008	2149	463	0	0
	Non-DOTS	0	475	0	0	120 814	0	0	0	0	7673	44 016	0	0	16	0	14 115	97
1999	DOTS	4	511	272	19 266	346 200	3	192	93	0	5831	40 800	253	23 936	2437	0	0	0
	Non-DOTS	0	562	0	0	113 969	0	0	0	0	1256	0	0	0	0	0	14 908	66
2000	DOTS	3	490	307	18 891	348 436	1	144	59	54	6011	15 397	210	0	1617	449	15 057	75
	Non-DOTS	0	553	0	0	114 937	0	0	0	0	1567	23 987	0	21 782	617	0	0	0
2001	DOTS	0	485	216	19 170	362 172	2	183	45	63	5907	17 809	189	0	1618	465	14 830	58
	Non-DOTS	3	495	0	0	123 049	0	0	0	0	1355	17 680	0	37 268	764	0	0	0

TABLE 13

Trend in tuberculosis notification (number of new smear-positives) in DOTS and non-DOTS areas, 1998–2001

Year		American Samoa	Australia	Brunei Darussalam	Cambodia	China	Cook Islands	Fiji	French Polynesia	Guam	Hong Kong, China	Japan	Kiribati	Republic of Korea	Lao PDR	Macao, China	Malaysia	N. Mariana Islands
1998	DOTS	6	116	0	13 865	191 290	1	74	34	0	0	0	50	10 359	1494	226	0	0
	non-DOTS	0	87	0	0	23 172	0	0	0	0	1869	11 935	0	0	14	0	7802	26
1999	DOTS	3	153	102	15 744	188 525	0	65	33	0	1566	12 909	59	9559	1719	0	0	0
	non-DOTS	0	133			23 901	0	0	0	0	0	0	0	0	0	0	7960	15
2000	DOTS	2	122	84	14 822	191 280	0	62	29	42	1517	4415	54	0	1526	133	8156	27
	non-DOTS	0	129	0	0	22 486	0	0	0	0	423	7438	0	8216	0	0	0	0
2001	DOTS	0	99	95	14 361	188 480	2	73	24	47	1425	5709	64	0	1533	157	8309	19
	non-DOTS	2	129	0	0	24 286	0	0	0	0	428	5699	0	11 805	0	0	0	0

Marshall Islands	Micronesia, FS	Mongolia	Nauru	New Caledonia	New Zealand	Niue	Palau	Papua New Guinea	Philippines	Pitcairn Islands	Samoa	Singapore	Solomon Islands	Tokelau	Tonga	Tuvalu	Vanuatu	Viet Nam	Wallis and Futuna	WPR total	%
																				839 142	
0	0	2725	0	102	0	1	15	2845	18 286	0	22	0	295	0	30	0		84 599	0	496 000	59
49	138	190	0	0	367	0	0	8446	141 580	0	0	2120	0	0	0	18	178	2850	0	343 142	41
																				823 421	
42	102	3348	0	0	0	0	32	1214	31 825	0	31	1654	289	0	22	0	86	88 426	0	566 869	69
0	0	0	0	0	348	2	0	10 975	113 982	0	0	0	0	0	0	0	31	453	0	256 552	31
																				806 970	
34	91	3109	4	0	344	0	0	2534	96 371	0	43	590	303	0	24	0	105	89 792	0	600 545	74
0	0	0	0	86	0	0	0	9587	32 124	0	0	1138	0	0	0	0	47	0	0	206 425	26
																				811 263	
56	95	3526	3	0	89	0	0	3470	107 133	0	22	749	292	0	11	0	121	90 679	0	629 458	78
0	0	0	0	64	288	0	0	0	0	0	0	787	0	0	0	0	52	0	0	181 805	22

Marshall Islands	Micronesia, FS	Mongolia	Nauru	New Caledonia	New Zealand	Niue	Palau	Papua New Guinea	Philippines	Pitcairn Islands	Samoa	Singapore	Solomon Islands	Tokelau	Tonga	Tuvalu	Vanuatu	Viet Nam	Wallis and Futuna	WPR total	%
																				393 257	
0	0	1213	0	30	0	0	7	418	10 292	0	7	0	140	0	16	0	0	53 147	0	282 785	72
11	28	143	0	0	81	0	0	1689	61 371	0	0	480	0	0	0	0	38	1726	0	110 472	28
																				393 802	
17	16	1513	0	0	0	0	20	254	20 477	0	17	465	93	0	10	0	24	53 561	0	306 904	78
0	0	0	0	0	69	1	0	1660	52 896	0	0	0	0	0	0	0	19	244	0	86 898	22
																				385 434	
11	15	1389	4	0	74	0	0	403	49 991	0	13	105	109	0	15	0	26	53 169	0	327 595	85
0	0	0	0	38	0	0	0	1864	17 065	0	0	143	0	0	0	0	37	0	0	57 839	15
																				379 060	
15	8	1631	2	0	21	0	0	462	59 341	0	12	175	118	0	8	0	46	54 202	0	336 438	89
0	0	0	0	34	47	0	0	0	0	0	0	182	0	0	0	0	10	0	0	42 622	11

TABLE 14

Trend in tuberculosis notification (rate for all types) in DOTS and non-DOTS areas, 1998–2001

		American Samoa	Australia	Brunei Darussalam	Cambodia	China	Cook Islands	Fiji	French Polynesia	Guam	Hong Kong, China	Japan	Kiribati	Republic of Korea	Lao PDR	Macao, China	Malaysia
1998	Population x 1000	63	18 445	313	10 751	1 255 091	20	822	227	161	6671	125 920	83	46 115	5358	440	21 450
	DOTS	9.5	2.3	0.0	157.6	26.8	10.0	20.2	46.3	0.0	0.0	0.0	332.5	65.1	40.1	105.2	0.0
	Non-DOTS	0.0	2.6	0.0	0.0	9.6	0.0	0.0	0.0	0.0	115.0	35.0	0.0	0.0	0.3	0.0	65.8
1999	Population x 1000	64	18 641	320	10 981	1 265 979	20	834	231	164	6729	126 187	85	46 505	5525	440	21 877
	DOTS	6.3	2.7	85.0	175.4	27.3	15.0	23.0	40.3	0.0	86.7	32.3	297.6	51.5	44.1	0.0	0.0
	Non-DOTS	0.0	3.0	0.0	0.0	9.0	0.0	0.0	0.0	0.0	18.7	0.0	0.0	0.0	0.0	0.0	68.1
2000	Population x 1000	68	19 138	328	13 104	1 275 133	20	814	233	155	6860	127 096	83	46 740	5279	444	22 218
	DOTS	4.4	2.6	93.5	144.2	27.3	5.1	17.7	25.3	34.8	87.6	12.1	253.3	0.0	30.6	101.1	67.8
	Non-DOTS	0.0	2.9	0.0	0.0	9.0	0.0	0.0	0.0	0.0	22.8	18.9	0.0	46.6	11.7	0.0	0.0
2001	Population x 1000	70	19 338	335	13 441	1 284 972	20	823	237	158	6961	127 335	84	47 069	5403	449	22 633
	DOTS	0.0	2.5	64.5	142.6	28.2	10.1	22.2	19.0	39.8	84.9	14.0	224.9	0.0	29.9	103.7	65.5
	Non-DOTS	4.3	2.6	0.0	0.0	9.6	0.0	0.0	0.0	0.0	19.5	13.9	0.0	79.2	14.1	0.0	0.0

TABLE 15

Trend in tuberculosis notification (rate for new smear-positives) in DOTS and non-DOTS areas, 1998–2001

		American Samoa	Australia	Brunei Darussalam	Cambodia	China	Cook Islands	Fiji	French Polynesia	Guam	Hong Kong, China	Japan	Kiribati	Republic of Korea	Lao PDR	Macao, China	Malaysia
1998	Population x 1000	63	18 445	313	10 751	1 255 091	20	822	227	161	6671	125920	83	46 115	5358	440	21 450
	DOTS	9.5	0.6	0.0	129.0	15.2	5.0	9.0	15.0	0.0	0.0	0.0	60.2	22.5	27.9	51.4	0.0
	Non-DOTS	0.0	0.5	0.0	0.0	1.8	0.0	0.0	0.0	0.0	28.0	9.5	0.0	0.0	0.3	0.0	36.4
1999	Population x 1000	64	18 641	320	10 981	1 265 979	20	834	231	164	6729	126187	85	46 505	5525	440	21 877
	DOTS	4.7	0.8	31.9	143.4	14.9	0.0	7.8	14.3	0.0	23.3	10.2	69.4	20.6	31.1	0.0	0.0
	Non-DOTS	0.0	0.7	0.0	0.0	1.9	0.0	0.0	0.0	0.0	0.0	0.0	0.0	0.0	0.0	0.0	36.4
2000	Population x 1000	68	19 138	328	13 104	1 275 133	20	814	233	155	6860	127096	83	46 740	5279	444	22 218
	DOTS	3.0	0.6	25.6	113.1	15.0	0.0	7.6	12.4	27.1	22.1	3.5	65.1	0.0	28.9	29.9	36.7
	Non-DOTS	0.0	0.7	0.0	0.0	1.8	0.0	0.0	0.0	0.0	6.2	5.9	0.0	17.6	0.0	0.0	0.0
2001	Population x 1000	70	19 338	335	13 441	1 284 972	20	823	237	158	6961	127335	84	47 069	5403	449	22 633
	DOTS	0.0	0.5	28.4	106.8	14.7	10.1	8.9	10.1	29.7	20.5	4.5	76.1	0.0	28.4	35.0	36.7
	Non-DOTS	2.9	0.7	0.0	0.0	1.9	0.0	0.0	0.0	0.0	6.1	4.5	0.0	25.1	0.0	0.0	0.0

N. Mariana Islands	Marshall Islands	Micronesia, FS	Mongolia	Nauru	New Caledonia	New Zealand	Niue	Palau	Papua New Guinea	Philippines	Pitcairn Islands	Samoa	Singapore	Solomon Islands	Tokelau	Tonga	Tuvalu	Vanuatu	Viet Nam	Wallis and Futuna	WPR total
70	61	134	2624	11	206	3680	2	17	4602	72 164	0	170	3491	417	2	99	10	182	77 896	14	1 657 782
0.0	0.0	0.0	103.8	0.0	49.5	0.0	50.0	88.2	61.8	25.3		12.9	0.0	70.7	0.0	30.3	0.0	0.0	108.6	0.0	29.9
138.6	80.3	103.0	7.2	0.0	0.0	10.0	0.0	0.0	183.5	196.2		0.0	60.7	0.0	0.0	0.0	13.0	97.8	3.7	0.0	20.7
74	63	137	2680	11	210	3719	2	18	4706	73 601	0	172	3541	460	2	100	10	187	79 228	14	1 673 517
0.0	66.7	74.5	124.9	0.0	0.0	0.0	0.0	177.8	25.8	43.2		18.0	46.7	62.8	0.0	22.0	0.0	46.0	111.6	0.0	33.9
89.2	0.0	0.0	0.0	0.0	0.0	9.4	100.0	0.0	233.2	154.9		0.0	0.0	0.0	0.0	0.0	0.0	16.6	0.6	0.0	15.3
73	51	123	2533	12	215	3778	2	19	4809	75 653	0	159	4018	447	1	99	10	197	78 137	14	1 688 065
103.0	66.5	74.1	122.7	32.7	0.0	9.1	0.0	0.0	52.7	127.4		27.1	14.7	67.7	0.0	24.2	0.0	53.4	114.9	0.0	35.6
0.0	0.0	0.0	0.0	0.0	39.9	0.0	0.0	0.0	199.3	42.5		0.0	28.3	0.0	0.0	0.0	0.0	23.9	0.0	0.0	12.2
76	52	126	2559	13	220	3808	2	20	4920	77 131	0	159	4108	463	1	99	10	202	79 175	15	1 702 484
76.4	108.1	75.5	137.8	24.0	0.0	2.3	0.0	0.0	70.5	138.9		13.8	18.2	63.1	0.0	11.1	0.0	59.9	114.5	0.0	37.0
0.0	0.0	0.0	0.0	0.0	29.1	7.6	0.0	0.0	0.0	0.0		0.0	19.2	0.0	0.0	0.0	0.0	25.8	0.0	0.0	10.7

N. Mariana Islands	Marshall Islands	Micronesia, FS	Mongolia	Nauru	New Caledonia	New Zealand	Niue	Palau	Papua New Guinea	Philippines	Pitcairn Islands	Samoa	Singapore	Solomon Islands	Tokelau	Tonga	Tuvalu	Vanuatu	Viet Nam	Wallis and Futuna	WPR total
70	61	134	2624	11	206	3680	2	17	4602	72 164	0	170	3491	417	2	99	10	182	77 896	14	1 657 782
0.0	0.0	0.0	46.2	0.0	14.6	0.0	0.0	41.2	9.1	14.3		4.1	0.0	33.6	0.0	16.2	0.0	0.0	68.2	0.0	17.1
37.1	18.0	20.9	5.4	0.0	0.0	2.2	0.0	0.0	36.7	85.0		0.0	13.7	0.0	0.0	0.0	0.0	20.9	2.2	0.0	6.7
74	63	137	2680	11	210	3719	2	18	4706	73 601	0	172	3541	460	2	100	10	187	79 228	14	1 673 517
0.0	27.0	11.7	56.5	0.0	0.0	0.0	0.0	111.1	5.4	27.8		9.9	13.1	20.2	0.0	10.0	0.0	12.8	67.6	0.0	18.3
20.3	0.0	0.0	0.0	0.0	0.0	1.9	50.0	0.0	35.3	71.9		0.0	0.0	0.0	0.0	0.0	0.0	10.2	0.3	0.0	5.2
73	51	123	2533	12	215	3778	2	19	4809	75 653	0	159	4018	447	1	99	10	197	78 137	14	1 688 065
37.1	21.5	12.2	54.8	32.7	0.0	2.0	0.0	0.0	8.4	66.1		8.2	2.6	24.4	0.0	15.1	0.0	13.2	68.0	0.0	19.4
0.0	0.0	0.0	0.0	0.0	17.7	0.0	0.0	0.0	38.8	22.6		0.0	3.6	0.0	0.0	0.0	0.0	18.8	0.0	0.0	3.4
76	52	126	2559	13	220	3808	2	20	4920	77 131	0	159	4108	463	1	99	10	202	79 175	15	1 702 484
25.0	28.9	6.4	63.7	16.0	0.0	0.6	0.0	0.0	9.4	76.9		7.6	4.3	25.5	0.0	8.0	0.0	22.8	68.5	0.0	19.8
0.0	0.0	0.0	0.0	0.0	15.5	1.2	0.0	0.0	0.0	0.0		0.0	4.4	0.0	0.0	0.0	0.0	5.0	0.0	0.0	2.5

TABLE 16

Treatment outcome of new smear-positive cases registered in 2000 in DOTS areas

| Country | Registered | Not evaluated (%) | Outcomes of treatment (%) | | | | | | Treatment success |
			Cured	Completed treatment	Defaulted	Failed	Died	Transferred out	
American Samoa	0								
Australia	114	5.3	19.3	54.4	1.8	0.0	7.9	11.4	73.7
Brunei Darussalam	84	0.0	41.7	21.4	3.6	0.0	16.7	16.7	63.1
Cambodia	14 775	0.0	87.8	3.5	3.9	0.3	3.6	0.8	91.4
China	191 280	1.8	94.6	0.0	0.8	1.0	1.0	0.9	94.6
Cook Islands	0								
Fiji	62	0.0	80.6	4.8	8.1	0.0	4.8	1.6	85.5
French Polynesia	62	0.0	0.0	96.8	0.0	1.6	1.6	0.0	96.8
Guam	43	0.0	93.0	0.0	0.0	0.0	7.0	0.0	93.0
Hong Kong, China	1517	0.0	70.3	5.3	4.3	8.0	3.9	8.2	75.6
Japan	4984	12.7	47.2	22.5	2.0	5.5	10.0	0.0	69.7
Kiribati	54	0.0	83.3	7.4	0.0	1.9	7.4	0.0	90.7
Republic of Korea	0								
Lao PDR	1392	0.0	72.8	8.7	8.5	0.4	6.8	2.8	81.5
Macao, China	160	0.0	81.3	8.1	4.4	0.0	5.6	0.6	89.4
Malaysia	0								
N. Mariana Islands	27	0.0	81.5	0.0	0.0	0.0	0.0	18.5	81.5
Marshall Islands	11	0.0	63.6	27.3	9.1	0.0	0.0	0.0	90.9
Micronesia, FS	14	0.0	92.9	0.0	0.0	0.0	7.1	0.0	92.9
Mongolia	1389	0.1	83.2	3.7	4.2	3.3	2.7	2.8	86.8
Nauru	0								
New Caledonia	0								
New Zealand	14	50.0	21.4	28.6	0.0	0.0	0.0	0.0	50.0
Niue	0								
Palau									
Papua New Guinea	422	4.7	38.6	24.2	25.6	0.5	2.4	4.0	62.8
Philippines	50 196	0.1	72.6	15.2	5.8	1.2	2.3	2.8	87.8
Pitcairn Islands									
Samoa	13	0.0	84.6	7.7	0.0	0.0	7.7	0.0	92.3
Singapore	105	0.0	0.0	84.8	7.6	1.0	6.7	0.0	84.8
Solomon Islands	118	0.0	66.1	26.3	6.8	0.0	0.8	0.0	92.4
Tokelau	0								
Tonga	15	0.0	93.3	0.0	0.0	6.7	0.0	0.0	93.3
Tuvalu									
Vanuatu	26	0.0	76.9	11.5	3.8	0.0	7.7	0.0	88.5
Viet Nam	53 169	0.1	89.9	2.2	1.8	1.0	3.1	1.9	92.1
Wallis and Futuna									
Total	**320 046**	**1.3**	**88.9**	**3.5**	**2.0**	**1.1**	**1.9**	**1.4**	**92.3**

TABLE 17

Treatment outcome of new smear-positive cases registered in 2000 in non-DOTS areas

Country	Registered	Not evaluated (%)	Outcomes of treatment (%)						Treatment success
			Cured	Completed treatment	Defaulted	Failed	Died	Transferred out	
American Samoa	2	0.0	0.0	100.0	0.0	0.0	0.0	0.0	100.0
Australia	124	14.5	33.9	37.1	3.2	0.0	9.7	1.6	71.0
Brunei Darussalam									
Cambodia									
China	22 486	2.9	81.3	0.0	4.0	7.4	1.6	2.8	81.3
Cook Islands									
Fiji									
French Polynesia									
Guam									
Hong Kong, China	423	78.3	2.4	5.0	1.4	0.0	11.1	1.9	7.3
Japan	5364	74.0	13.8	8.9	0.4	2.2	0.7	0.0	22.7
Kiribati									
Republic of Korea	3231	0.8	80.9	1.6	3.1	1.3	1.6	10.7	82.5
Lao PDR	62	0.0	53.2	11.3	19.4	1.6	12.9	1.6	64.5
Macao, China									
Malaysia									
N. Mariana Islands									
Marshall Islands									
Micronesia, FS									
Mongolia									
Nauru	4	25.0	25.0	0.0	0.0	0.0	0.0	50.0	25.0
New Caledonia	45	0.0	33.3	55.6	2.2	0.0	8.9	0.0	88.9
New Zealand	59	74.6	1.7	23.7	0.0	0.0	0.0	0.0	25.4
Niue									
Palau									
Papua New Guinea	6165	0.0	0.0	67.3	14.4	5.3	3.6	9.4	67.3
Philippines									
Pitcairn Islands									
Samoa									
Singapore	137	0.0	0.0	61.3	19.7	0.0	19.0	0.0	61.3
Solomon Islands									
Tokelau									
Tonga									
Tuvalu									
Vanuatu	37	100.0	0.0	0.0	0.0	0.0	0.0	0.0	0.0
Viet Nam									
Wallis and Futuna									
Total	38 139	13.3	57.0	12.8	5.2	5.6	2.0	4.1	69.8

TABLE 18

Treatment outcome of re-treatment cases registered in 2000 in DOTS areas

Country	Registered	Not evaluated (%)	Outcomes of treatment (%)						
			Cured	Completed treatment	Defaulted	Failed	Died	Transferred out	Treatment success
American Samoa									
Australia	7	0.0	0.0	85.7	0	0	0	14.3	85.7
Brunei Darussalam									
Cambodia	827	0.0	85.4	4.6	0	0	0	0.1	90.0
China	43 252	8.0	86.5	2.2	0	0	0	0.4	88.6
Cook Islands									
Fiji									
French Polynesia									
Guam									
Hong Kong, China	218	0.0	26.6	26.1	0	0	0	7.8	52.8
Japan	605	13.1	46.4	20.8	0	0	0	0.0	67.3
Kiribati	9	0.0	88.9	0.0	0	0	0	0.0	88.9
Republic of Korea									
Lao PDR	51	0.0	51.0	9.8	0	0	0	2.0	60.8
Macao, China	37	0.0	67.6	16.2	0	0	0	0.0	83.8
Malaysia									
N. Mariana Islands									
Marshall Islands									
Micronesia, FS	20	0.0	25.0	60.0	0	0	0	0.0	85.0
Mongolia	126	0.8	57.1	14.3	0	0	0	4.8	71.4
Nauru									
New Caledonia									
New Zealand	8	50.0	0.0	50.0	0	0	0	0.0	50.0
Niue									
Palau									
Papua New Guinea	68	2.9	29.4	35.3	0	0	0	5.9	64.7
Philippines									
Pitcairn Islands									
Samoa									
Singapore									
Solomon Islands	3	0.0	0.0	100.0	0	0	0	0.0	100.0
Tokelau									
Tonga	1	0.0	100.0	0.0	0	0	0	0.0	100.0
Tuvalu									
Vanuatu	5	0.0	100.0	0.0	0	0	0	0.0	100.0
Viet Nam	8806	3.5	74.0	4.7	0	0	0	3.3	78.7
Wallis and Futuna									
Total	**54 043**	**7.2**	**83.5**	**3.0**	**1.3**	**2.0**	**2.2**	**0.9**	**86.6**

TABLE 19

Treatment outcome of re-treatment cases registered in 2000 in non-DOTS areas

Country	Registered	Not evaluated (%)	Outcomes of treatment (%)						
			Cured	Completed treatment	Defaulted	Failed	Died	Transferred out	Treatment success
American Samoa									
Australia	4	0.0	25.0	50.0	0	0	0	0.0	75.0
Brunei Darussalam									
Cambodia									
China									
Cook Islands									
Fiji									
French Polynesia									
Guam									
Hong Kong, China	13	0.0	23.1	7.7	0	0	1	7.7	30.8
Japan	564	70.6	15.2	9.4	0	0	0	0.0	24.6
Kiribati									
Republic of Korea	131	2.3	58.8	1.5	0	0	0	19.1	60.3
Lao PDR									
Macao, China									
Malaysia									
N. Mariana Islands									
Marshall Islands									
Micronesia									
Mongolia									
Nauru									
New Caledonia									
New Zealand	15	73.3	0.0	20.0	0	0	0	0.0	20.0
Niue									
Palau									
Papua New Guinea									
Philippines									
Pitcairn Islands									
Samoa									
Singapore									
Solomon Islands									
Tokelau									
Tonga									
Tuvalu									
Vanuatu	1	100.0	0.0	0.0	0	0	0	0.0	0.0
Viet Nam									
Wallis and Futuna									
Total	728	56.7	22.9	8.4	2.2	4.1	2.1	3.6	31.3

PART III

Charts

Chart 1
Notification of all cases (rate per 100 000) by country,
Western Pacific Region, 2001 34

Chart 2
Notification of new smear-positive cases (rate per 100 000) by country,
Western Pacific Region, 2001 35

Chart 3
Notification rate of new smear-positive cases by age and sex in DOTS areas,
Western Pacific Region, 2001 36

Chart 4
DOTS enrolment rate in high-burden countries,
Western Pacific Region, 2001 36

Chart 5
DOTS enrolment rate of new smear-positive cases in high-burden countries,
Western Pacific Region, 1997 and 2001 37

Chart 6
DOTS case detection rate of new smear-positive cases in high-burden countries,
Western Pacific Region, 2001 37

Chart 7
Treatment success of new smear-positive cases under DOTS in high-burden countries,
Western Pacific Region, 2001 38

Chart 8
DOTS progress in high-burden countries in the Western Pacific Region, 1998–2001 38

Charts

CHART 1

Notification of all cases (rate per 100 000) by country, Western Pacific Region, 2001

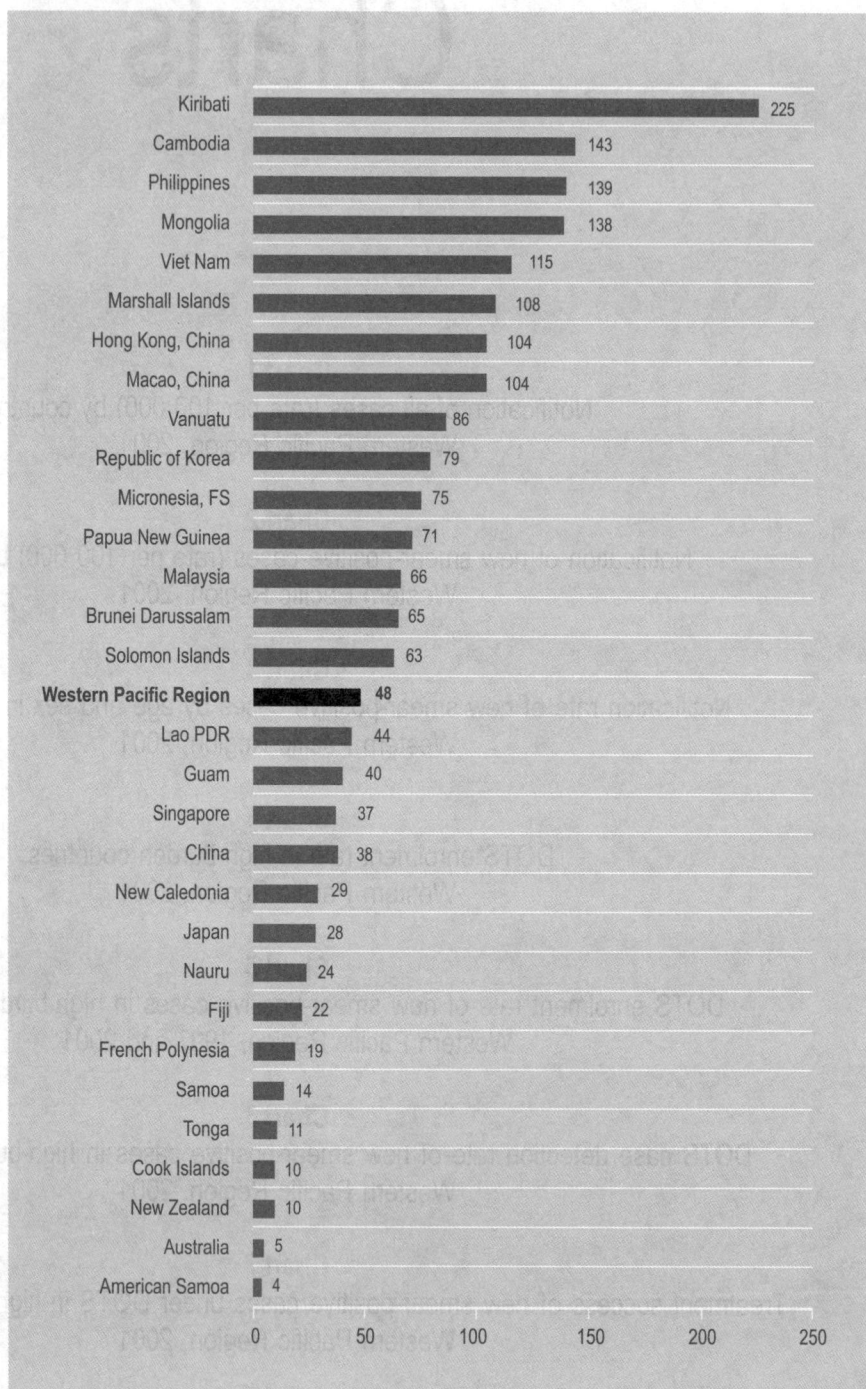

Country	Rate
Kiribati	225
Cambodia	143
Philippines	139
Mongolia	138
Viet Nam	115
Marshall Islands	108
Hong Kong, China	104
Macao, China	104
Vanuatu	86
Republic of Korea	79
Micronesia, FS	75
Papua New Guinea	71
Malaysia	66
Brunei Darussalam	65
Solomon Islands	63
Western Pacific Region	**48**
Lao PDR	44
Guam	40
Singapore	37
China	38
New Caledonia	29
Japan	28
Nauru	24
Fiji	22
French Polynesia	19
Samoa	14
Tonga	11
Cook Islands	10
New Zealand	10
Australia	5
American Samoa	4

CHART 2

Notification of new smear-positive cases (rate per 100 000) by country, Western Pacific Region, 2001

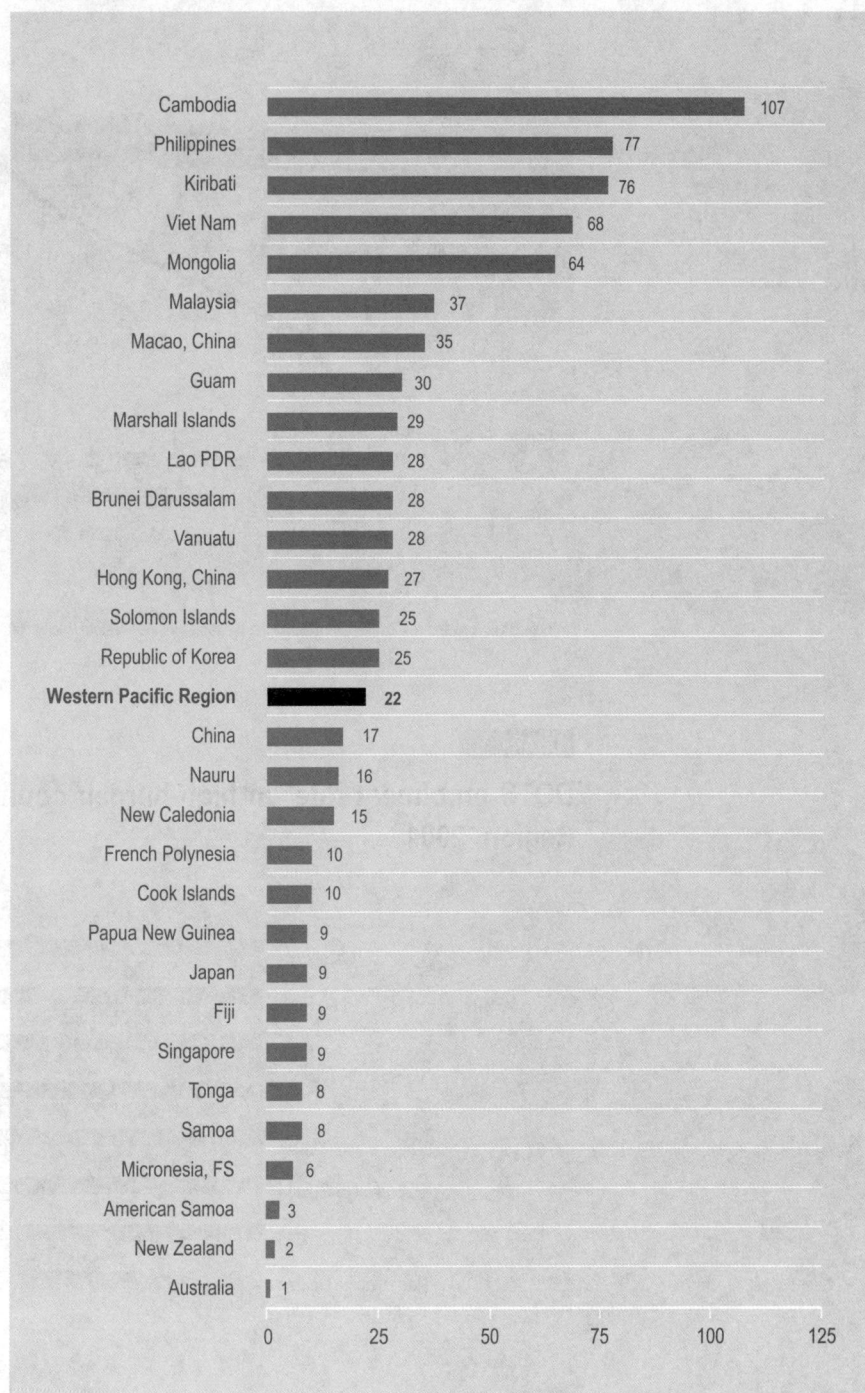

Country	Rate
Cambodia	107
Philippines	77
Kiribati	76
Viet Nam	68
Mongolia	64
Malaysia	37
Macao, China	35
Guam	30
Marshall Islands	29
Lao PDR	28
Brunei Darussalam	28
Vanuatu	28
Hong Kong, China	27
Solomon Islands	25
Republic of Korea	25
Western Pacific Region	**22**
China	17
Nauru	16
New Caledonia	15
French Polynesia	10
Cook Islands	10
Papua New Guinea	9
Japan	9
Fiji	9
Singapore	9
Tonga	8
Samoa	8
Micronesia, FS	6
American Samoa	3
New Zealand	2
Australia	1

CHART 3

Notification rate of new smear-positive cases by age and sex* in DOTS areas, Western Pacific Region, 2001

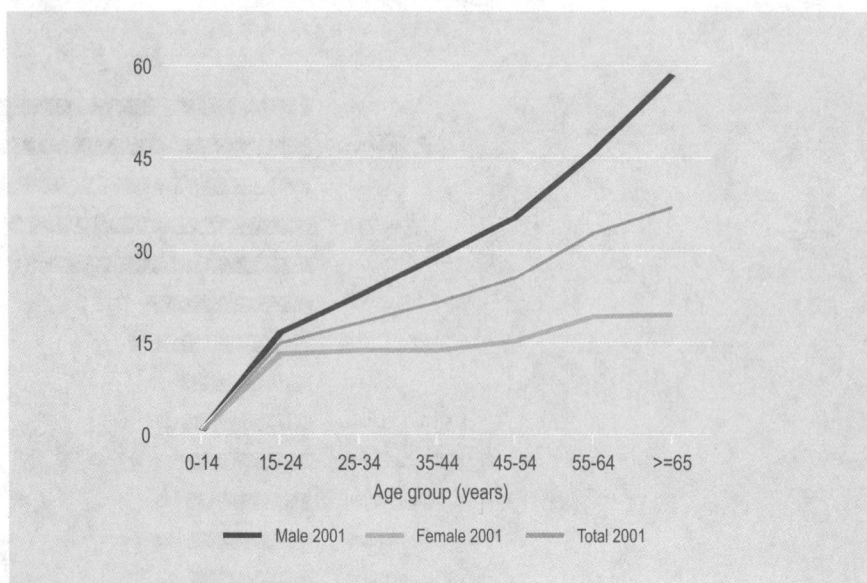

*Population by age and sex is taken from Demographic Tables for the Western Pacific Region, 2000–2005.

CHART 4

DOTS enrolment rate* in high-burden countries, Western Pacific Region, 2001

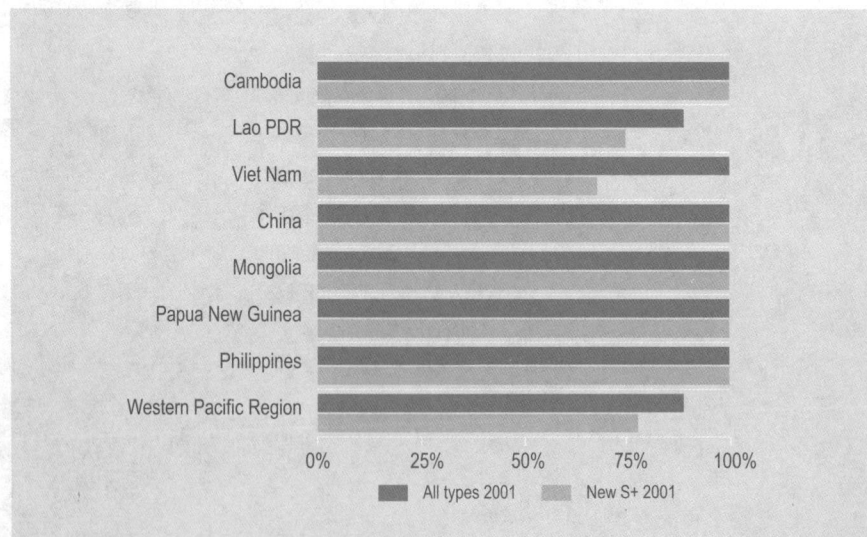

*Population of notified cases enroled under DOTS strategy out of all notified cases.

CHART 5

DOTS enrolment rate* of new smear-positive cases in high-burden countries, Western Pacific Region, 1997 and 2001

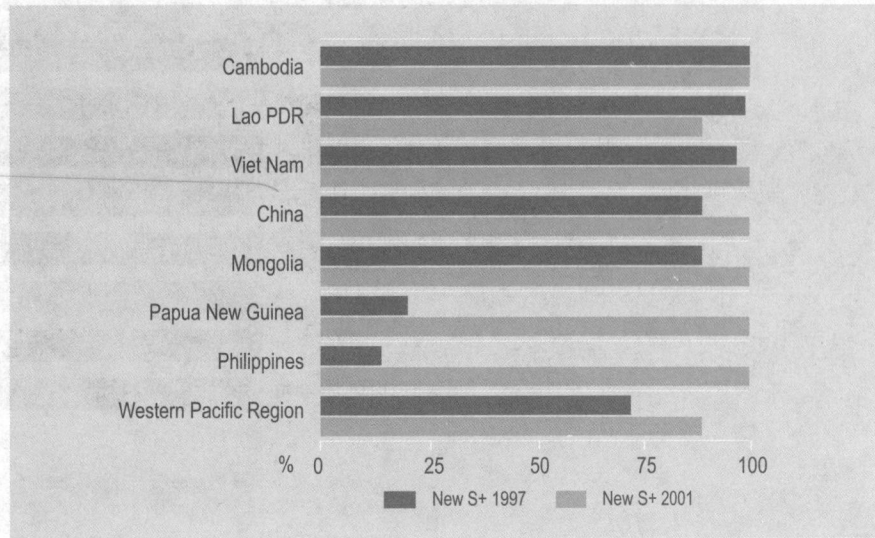

*Population of notified cases enroled under DOTS strategy out of all notified cases.

CHART 6

DOTS case detection rate of new smear-positive cases in high-burden countries, Western Pacific Region, 2001

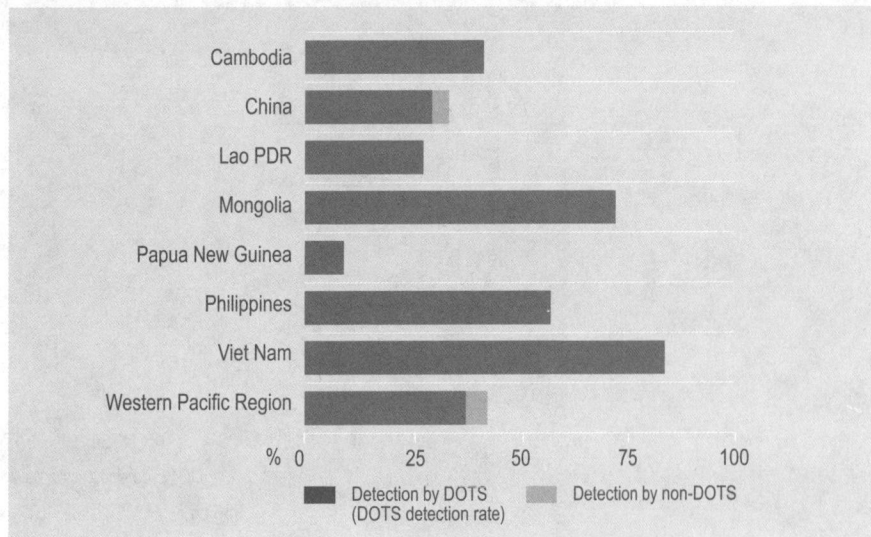

CHART 7

Treatment success of new smear-positive cases under DOTS in high-burden countries, Western Pacific Region, 2001

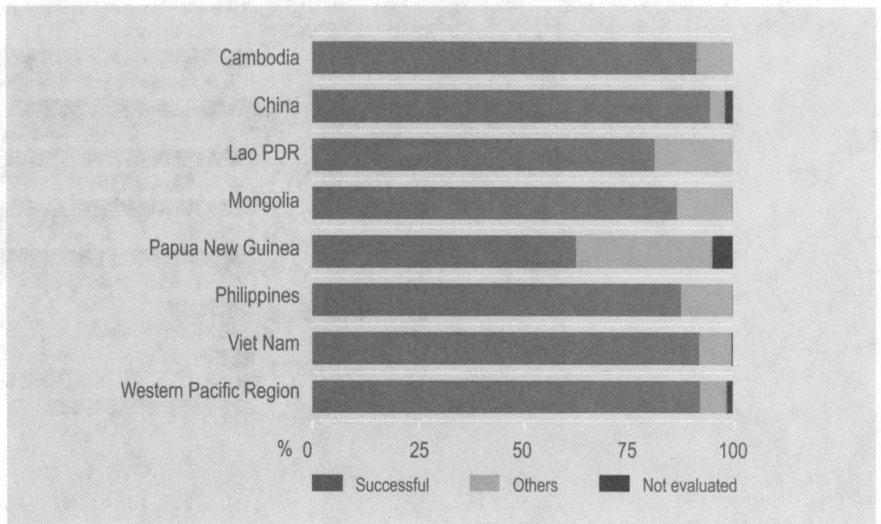

CHART 8

DOTS progress in high-burden countries in the Western Pacific Region, 1998–2001

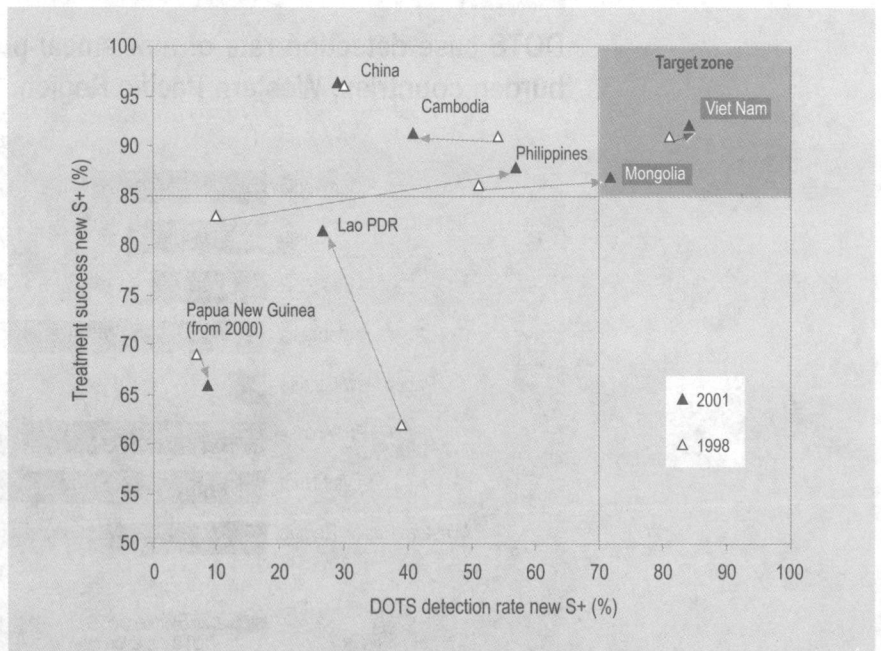

Annexes

Annex 1
Profiles of high-burden countries in the Western Pacific Region 40

Annex 2
Definitions 48

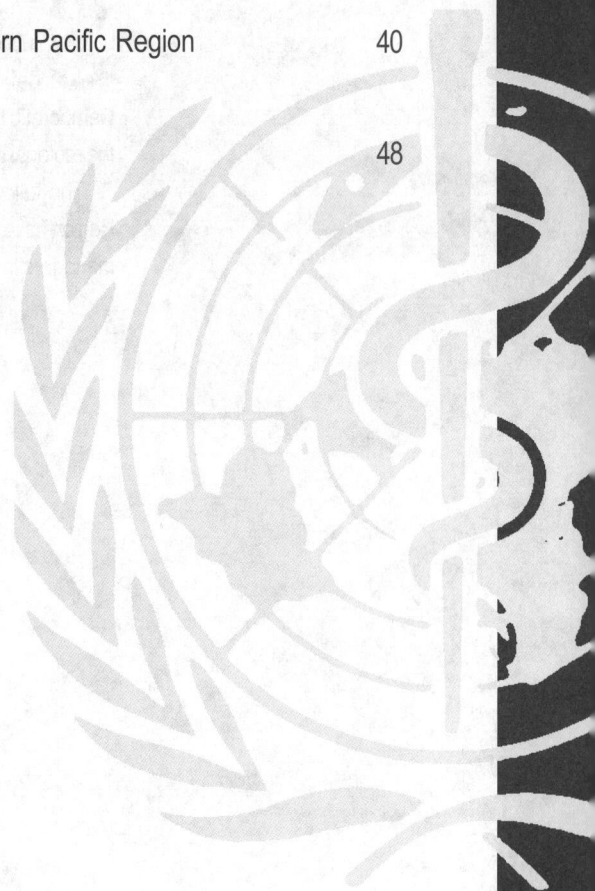

Profiles of high-burden countries in the Western Pacific Region

S even countries in the Region have been identified as having a high burden of tuberculosis. Cambodia, China, the Philippines and Viet Nam are among the 22 globally defined high-burden countries (based on estimated incidence); the Lao People's Democratic Republic, Mongolia and Papua New Guinea are defined as high-burden countries in the regional context.

The following country profiles for the seven high-burden countries in the Western Pacific Region have been updated using information provided during the last regional meeting of the NTP managers in Cebu, Philippines (December 2002).

DOTS enrolment and treatment success rates are high. Increased case detection is expected in the coming year following expansion of DOTS to more operational districts.

TABLE A1

Key indicators for tuberculosis control, 1998–2001

Key Indicators	1998	2001
Total population x 1000	10 715	13 441
Notification all cases	16 946	19 170
Notification new S+	13 865	14 361
New S+ out of all cases, %	82	75
Detection rate all cases, %	24	24
Detection rate new S+, %	54	41
Population with access to DOTS, %	100	100
DOTS enrolment rate (new S+, %)	98	98
DOTS case detection rate (new S+, %)	53	40
Treatment success under DOTS (new S+, %)	91	91
Prevalence of HIV infection among tuberculosis cases, %	5.2 (1997)	8.4 (2002)

Cambodia

is ranked the 20th high burden country for tuberculosis globally and fourth in the Region (by estimated incidence of all cases). The NTP has set up DOTS in all 77 operational districts in 145 tuberculosis units and in 381 health centres (40%) at village level, in order to monitor the continuation phase of treatment. DOTS enrolment and treatment success rates are high. Increased case detection is expected in the coming year following expansion of DOTS to more operational districts. Prevalence of HIV infection among tuberculosis patients is a major concern and has increased, from 6% in 2000 to 8.4% in 2002 (in a sentinel group of 2358 tuberculosis patients in 21 provinces, HIV/AIDS Sentinel Surveillance 2002, NCHADS, Cambodia).

DOTS Progress	DOTS started in 1994
(1) Political commitment	Clear policies, guidelines and plans in line with DOTS
	Regular Interagency Coordinating Committee meetings
	90% of management posts filled
(2) Diagnosis by microscopy	Smear microscopy available in 145 tuberculosis units
	Culture and drug sensitivity testing at central level
	Quality assurance at central and district level
	90% of diagnostic centres provide good quality services
(3) DOT and tuberculosis drugs	Available > 95% of the time
	98% DOTS enrolment of new smear-positive cases
	In all province and district hospitals and 40% of the health centres
(4) Monitoring	Training and supervision according to plan
	Reporting from all tuberculosis units

Multidrug resistance (combined resistance to at least rifampicin and isoniazide) was found to be high in China, ranging from 2.9% to 5.3% of newly detected cases in three provinces.

TABLE A2

Key indicators for tuberculosis control, 1998–2001

Key Indicators	1998	2001
Total population x 1000	1 255 697	1 284 972
Notification all cases	457 349	485 221
Notification new S+	214 462	212 766
New S+ out of all cases, %	47	44
Detection rate all cases, %	32	34
Detection rate new S+, %	33	33
Population with access to DOTS, %	64	68
DOTS enrolment rate (new S+, %)	74	75
DOTS case detection rate (new S+, %)	89	89
Treatment success under DOTS (new S+, %)	30	29
Treatment success new S+, % DOTS (non-DOTS)	96	96 (81)
Primary multidrug resistant tuberculosis (new S+, %)		
Guangdong	—	(2000) 5.3
Zhejiang		4.3
Shandong		2.9

China

has the second highest tuberculosis burden globally and is ranked highest in the Region with 70% of estimated all cases and 61% of all notified cases in 2001. The case detection rate for new smear-positive cases (out of estimated cases) was 33%. About 68% of the population has access to DOTS. Treatment success was 82% for new smear-positive cases (cohort 2000 in DOTS areas). A new NTP started in 2002 in 31 provinces (after the World Bank Health V project and Ministry of Health projects terminated in 2001). Multidrug resistance (combined resistance to at least rifampicin and isoniazide) was found to be high in China, ranging from 2.9% to 5.3% of newly detected cases in three provinces (2000). A joint monitoring mission in November 2002 identified several major constraints: insufficient human resources at central and provincial levels, inadequate financial support from prefectures/counties, lack of budgeted planning, weak drugs procurement and management capacity, and difficulty maintaining quality of DOTS in the context of rapid programme expansion and ensuring complementary funding from different sources.

DOTS Progress	DOTS started in 1991
(1) Political commitment	Tuberculosis manual and guidelines in line with DOTS ICC meeting Support from CIDA, DFB, GFATM, JICA, KNCV, WB, WHO 2003 DOTS expansion plan available
(2) Diagnosis by microscopy	Smear microscopy available in 31 provinces, 321 prefectures and 1857 counties (65%) Culture available in 31 provinces, 216 prefectures and 230 counties (8%) Drug sensitivity testing in 15 provinces and 21 prefectures Quality assurance in all microscopy centres Adequate quality in 70–90% of diagnosis centres
(3) DOT and tuberculosis drugs	89% DOTS enrolment of new smear-positive cases Available > 95% of the time
(4) Monitoring	Training, supervision according to plan, joint monitoring mission in five provinces in November 2002 Reporting <80% of tuberculosis units

Full DOTS coverage is expected by the end of 2003. Also, DOTS will be decentralized in health posts at village level in three pilot provinces.

TABLE A3

Key indicators for tuberculosis control, 1998–2001

Key Indicators	1998	2001
Total population x 1000	5163	5403
Notification all cases	2165	2382
Notification new S+	1508	1533
New S+ out of all cases, %	70	64
Detection rate all cases, %	25	19
Detection rate new S+, %	39	27
Population with access to DOTS, %	71	78
DOTS enrolment rate (new S+, %)	99	100
DOTS case detection rate (new S+, %)	39	26
Treatment success under DOTS (new S+, %)	62	82

The Lao People's Democratic Republic was ranked the fifth high-burden country for

tuberculosis in the Region in 2001. DOTS had started in 16 provinces and 92 districts by the end of 2002. The two remaining provinces (with 32 districts) will start DOTS in 2003. The case detection rate for smear-positive cases was 26% in 2001 with treatment success reaching 82%.

DOTS is implemented in the government hospital service, from central to district hospital level, in 163 DOTS units covering 74.5% of the population. Tuberculosis drugs are free for hospitalized patients (in government hospitals). DOTS is not extended to the private sector (clinics and pharmacies). Full DOTS coverage is expected by the end of 2003. Also, DOTS will be decentralized in health posts at village level in three pilot provinces.

DOTS Progress	DOTS started in 1995
(1) Political commitment	No ICC established, 2003 plan available
	50–80% of tuberculosis staff positions filled
	Tuberculosis manual and guidelines in line with DOTS strategy
(2) Diagnosis by microscopy	95% of laboratory technicians trained for tuberculosis
	Culture and drug sensitivity testing not available
	Quality assurance at central level and provinces in all centres by random sampling
	Adequate quality in 70–90% of diagnosis centres
(3) DOT and tuberculosis drugs	Available > 95% of the time
(4) Monitoring	100% DOTS enrolment of new smear-positive cases
	Training and supervision follow plans
	<80% of tuberculosis units report to the central level

Mongolia passed WHO targets for the first time in 2001, attaining a DOTS case detection rate of 72% and treatment success of 87% for new smear-positive cases.

TABLE A4

Key indicators for tuberculosis control, 1998–2001

Key Indicators	1998	2001
Total population x 1000	2579	2559
Notification all cases	2915	3526
Notification new S+	1356	1631
New S+ out of all cases, %	47	46
Detection rate all cases, %	55	70
Detection rate new S+, %	57	72
Population with access to DOTS, %	97	100
DOTS enrolment rate (new S+, %)	89	100
DOTS case detection rate (new S+, %)	51	72
Treatment success under DOTS (new S+, %)	86	87

Mongolia

was ranked the seventh highest burden country for tuberculosis in the Region in 2001. It passed WHO targets for the first time in 2001, attaining a DOTS case detection rate of 72% and treatment success of 87% for new smear-positive cases, two years after attaining full DOTS coverage (21 *aimags* and eight districts) in 1999. DOTS was also extended to all prisons in 1999 (with a cure rate of 65% in 2001). Next, the programme will be targeted towards developing mechanisms for implementing Global Fund support, increasing quality of DOTS in rural areas (by collaborating with poverty projects and involving family doctors) and strengthening the quality of laboratory services.

DOTS Progress	DOTS started in 1995
(1) Political commitment	2003 plan available
	Tuberculosis manual and guidelines in line with DOTS
	Regular Inter Agency Coordination Committee meetings
	Support from DANIDA extended up to 1994
	Global Fund
(2) Diagnosis by microscopy	Diagnosis centres are adequate
	Effective quality assessment system
	Adequate quality in > 90% of the diagnosis centres
(3) DOT and tuberculosis drugs	Operational guidelines are available in tuberculosis manual
	Drugs available 70–95% of the time
	100% DOTS enrolment of new smear-positive cases
(4) Monitoring	>80% of tuberculosis staff positions are filled
	Training plans available and implemented
	Supervision according to plan
	>80% of tuberculosis units are submitting reports

DOTS started in 1997 and covered eight provinces (18% of the population) by the end of 2002. In 2001, 3470 cases were notified in DOTS provinces.

TABLE A5

Key indicators for tuberculosis control, 1998–2001

Key Indicators	1998	2001
Total population x 1000	4599	4920
Notification all cases	11 291	3470
Notification new S+	2107	462
New S+ out of all cases, %	19	13
Detection rate all cases, %	98	29
Detection rate new S+, %	41	9
Population with access to DOTS %	9	13
DOTS enrolment rate (new S+, %)	20	100
DOTS case detection rate (new S+, %)	8	8
Treatment success under DOTS (new S+, %)	93	63
Primary multidrug resistance (2000)		1

Papua New Guinea was ranked as having the sixth highest burden of tuberculosis

in the Region in 2001. DOTS started in 1997 and covered eight provinces (18% of the population) by the end of 2002. In 2001, 3470 cases were notified in DOTS provinces through the tuberculosis quarterly reporting system. Also, 15 897 "on treatment" tuberculosis cases all types (including 1122 sputum positive cases) were reported through the monthly health information system from 571 health centres (non-DOTS provinces). Treatment success (new smear-positives, cohort 2000) was 63%.

The priorities are to strengthen programme management in the central and regional levels, expand DOTS in the 12 remaining provinces, improve funding from provinces and districts, upgrade laboratory services (providing refresher training for province laboratory staff, laboratory equipment and consumables, and development of quality assessment) and increase supervision from provinces to districts and from districts to below.

DOTS Progress	DOTS started in 1997
(1) Political commitment	Insufficient human resources in central unit
	2003 plan available
	Tuberculosis manual and guidelines in line with DOTS
	ICC was funded in 2002 and taken over by the Coordination
	Committee of the Global Fund
(2) Diagnosis by microscopy	Inadequate laboratory services with shortage of staff in periphery
	Quality assessment is not routinely carried out
	70 to 90 of the evaluated centers have satisfactory quality
(3) DOT and tuberculosis drugs	Operational guidelines are available in the new manual
	Drugs are available 70–95% of the time
	100% DOTS enrolment of new smear-positive cases
(4) Monitoring	Training plan is available and implemented in phases
	Supervision guidelines are not routinely used
	>80% of the tuberculosis units (in DOTS provinces) report to central level

DOTS started in 1996 and was rapidly expanded to cover 97% of the population. The DOTS case detection rate also rose rapidly to 57% in 2001.

TABLE A6

Key indicators for tuberculosis control, 1998–2001

Key Indicators	1998	2001
Total population x 1000	72 944	77 131
Notification all cases	159 866	107 133
Notification new S+	71 663	59 341
New S+ out of all cases, %	45	55
Detection rate all cases, %	70	46
Detection rate new S+, %	70	57
Population with access to DOTS, %	17	97
DOTS enrolment rate (new S+, %)	14	100
DOTS case detection rate (new S+, %)	10	57
Treatment success under DOTS (new S+, %)	83	88

The Philippines

was ranked as having the seventh highest tuberculosis burden globally and second in the Region in 2001. It reported 13% of all cases notified in the Region in 2001.

DOTS started in 1996 and was rapidly expanded to cover 97% of the population. The DOTS case detection rate also rose rapidly to 57% in 2001 (from only 10% in 1998), while the treatment success rate is 88%.

Smear microscopy is available in each rural health unit or municipality with one validation centre in each province or city. Tuberculosis reference laboratories (national and regional) can perform culture and drug sensitivity tests. Shortages of tuberculosis staff at the central and regional levels and training at province and hospital levels are major constraints. Delayed procurement and distribution of tuberculosis drugs are also a recurrent problem, resulting in drug shortages and absence of buffer stock. In municipalities, local government units may buy variable and budget-driven amounts of drugs (Category 3) for smear-negative or extrapulmonary cases. A Public-Private Mix DOTS pilot project aims at involving the private sector in DOTS.

DOTS Progress	DOTS started in 1996
(1) Political commitment	Strong central NTP unit (but shortage of staff)
	New Manual of Procedures diffused in line with DOTS
	Funding gap < 30%
	Provinces and municipalities have allocated funds for staffing
	Regular ICC meeting with partners
	Inadequate advocacy and promotion to increase demand
	Lack of involvement of the private sector
(2) Diagnosis by microscopy	Diagnosis centres adequate and well staffed
	Quality assessment system is in place but the laboratory network needs to be strengthened
(3) DOT and tuberculosis drugs	Operational guidelines are available in the new Manual of Procedures
	100% DOTS enrolment of new smear-positive cases
	Tuberculosis drugs subject to quality criteria
	Delayed procurement and delivery of drugs, available less than 70% of the time in one year
(4) Monitoring	Inadequate monitoring and supervision
	>80% of the tuberculosis units submit reports but with some delay

About 1% of
Viet Nam's
tuberculosis
patients were
infected by HIV,
although in some
provinces more
than 5% of
tuberculosis
cases were
due to HIV.

TABLE A7

Key indicators for tuberculosis control, 1998–2001

Key Indicators	1998	2001
Total population x 1000	77 562	79 175
Notification all cases	87 449	90 679
Notification new S+	54 873	54 202
New S+ out of all cases, %	63	60
Detection rate all cases, %	60	63
Detection rate new S+, %	83	84
Population with access to DOTS, %	96	100
DOTS enrolment rate (new S+, %)	97	100
DOTS case detection rate (new S+, %)	81	83
Treatment success under DOTS (new S+, %)	91	92
Prevalence of HIV infection among tuberculosis cases, %		1 (2000)
Primary multidrug resistance		

Viet Nam

was ranked 13th among the 22 highest burden countries globally (2000) and third in the Region, with 11% of all cases in 2001. About 1% of Viet Nam's tuberculosis patients were infected by HIV, although in some provinces more than 5% of tuberculosis cases were due to HIV (in 2000). Major constraints are low case detection in remote areas, fast development of the private sector, rapid turnover of staff in the context of health sector reforms, increased HIV prevalence among tuberculosis cases, and stigmatization of tuberculosis among health staff and the general public. NTP priorities are to improve the quality of DOTS in remote areas, step up tuberculosis education in the community, and coordinate and integrate tuberculosis control with other programmes (the HIV programme and the Expanded Programme of Immunization).

DOTS Progress	
(1) Political commitment	Strong NTP central unit, 2003 implementation plan available, NTP manual in line with DOTS, no funding gap, regular iCC meetings
(2) Diagnosis by microscopy	Microscopy services available and well staffed
	With effective quality assessment system, 70–90% of centres are of adequate quality
	Two National Reference Laboratories (culture, drug sensitivity testing, training, monitoring, research), 61 province laboratories (smear examination, culture, quality assessment, training, supervision) and 623 district laboratories (smear examination, quality assessment)
	Quality assessment by double reading, all positive and 10% negative
(3) DOT and tuberculosis drugs	Operational guidelines are available in the tuberculosis manual
	>80% of new smear-positives are under DOTS
	Tuberculosis drugs available, >95% with quality assessment
(4) Monitoring	Training plan and supervision guidelines are available and implemented, >80% of reporting units submit their reports

Definitions[6]

Definitions of tuberculosis cases

A case of tuberculosis: A patient in whom tuberculosis has been bacteriologically confirmed, or has been diagnosed by a clinician. Any person given treatment for tuberculosis should be recorded.

All types: The sum of new smear-positive pulmonary, relapse, new smear-negative pulmonary and extrapulmonary cases.

New smear-positive pulmonary: A patient who has never received treatment for tuberculosis or has taken anti-tuberculosis drugs for less than four weeks and who has one of the following:
- Two or more initial sputum smear examinations positive for acid fast bacilli (AFB); or
- one sputum examination positive for AFB plus radiographic abnormalities consistent with active pulmonary tuberculosis as determined by a treating medical officer; or
- one sputum specimen positive for AFB and at least one sputum specimen that is culture positive for AFB.

New smear-negative pulmonary: A case of pulmonary tuberculosis that does not meet the above definition for smear-positive tuberculosis:

Extrapulmonary tuberculosis: Tuberculosis of organs other than the lungs: e.g. pleura, lymph nodes, abdomen, genito-urinary tract, skin, joints and bones, meninges, etc. Diagnosis should be based on one culture-positive specimen, or histological or strong clinical evidence consistent with active extrapulmonary tuberculosis, followed by a decision by a clinician to treat with a full course of anti-tuberculosis chemotherapy. (A patient diagnosed with both pulmonary and extrapulmonary tuberculosis should be classified as a case of pulmonary tuberculosis.)

Retreatment cases: Relapses, failures and defaulters.

Relapse: A patient previously treated for tuberculosis and declared cured or treatment completed, who is later diagnosed with bacteriologically positive (culture smear) tuberculosis.

Definitions of treatment outcome

Cured: A patient who is sputum smear-negative in the last month of treatment and on at least one previous occasion.

Completed treatment: A patient who has completed treatment but who does not meet the criteria to be classified as a cure or a failure.

Treatment success: The sum of patients who are cured and those who have completed treatment.

---

[6] WHO, IUATLD, KNCV. Revised International Definitions in Tuberculosis Control. Int J Tuberc Lung Dis 2001; 5: 213–215.

Died: A patient who dies for any reason during the course of treatment.

Failure: A patient who is sputum smear-positive at five months or later during the course of treatment.

Defaulted: A patient who has interrupted treatment for two consecutive months or more.

Transferred out: A patient who has been transferred to another recording and reporting unit and for whom the treatment outcome is not known.

Not evaluated: Patients who did not have the treatment outcome evaluated.

Note: In countries where culture is current practice, patients can be classified as cured or a failure on the basis of culture results.

Indicators to assess treatment outcome

Cure rate: Proportion of cured cases out of all cases registered in a certain period (in 2000 in this report).

Treatment success rates: The sum of the proportion of patients who were cured and patients who completed treatment out of all cases registered in a certain period. The global target is a cure rate of 85% and a greater treatment success rate.

The cure rate and treatment success rate are expressed as a percentage of registered cases. The number of new cases registered for treatment in 2000 (reported in 2002) is compared to the number of cases notified as smear-positive in 2000 (reported in 2001). Differences may arise because NTPs do not compile data at the end of each calendar year, diagnoses may be incorrect, patients are lost between diagnosis and the start of treatment, or records are lost. Second, only a fraction of registered cases was evaluated for outcome. All registered cases should be evaluated. Third, data on the six standard, mutually exclusive outcomes of treatment are compiled. These figures are reported as percentages of all registered cases, so that the possible outcomes plus the fraction of cases not evaluated sum to 100%. When a country states the number of patients registered for treatment, but gives no outcomes, no result is reported rather than zero treatment success. Although treatment outcomes are expressed as percentages, they are referred to as rates. The six possible outcomes plus the fraction of cases not evaluated total 100%. If the number of registered cases is lower than the sum of the six outcomes or is missing, the denominator for treatment success will be the number evaluated or the number of smear-positive cases notified in the previous year, whichever is greater.

Case detection rate and DOTS detection rate

DOTS. The recommended strategy for tuberculosis control. It comprises

- government commitment to ensuring sustained, comprehensive tuberculosis control activities;
- case detection by sputum smear microscopy among symptomatic patients self-reporting to health services;
- standardized short-course chemotherapy using regimens of six to eight months, for at least all confirmed smear-positive cases. Good case management includes DOT during the intensive phase for all new sputum smear-positive cases, the continuation phase of rifampicin-containing regimens and the whole re-treatment regimen;
- a regular, uninterrupted drug supply of all essential anti-tuberculosis drugs; and
- a standardized recording and reporting system that allows assessment of case-finding and treatment results for each patient and of the tuberculosis control programme performance overall.

Targets for tuberculosis control were established by the World Health Assembly:
- to cure 85% of the sputum smear-positive tuberculosis cases detected; and
- to detect 70% of the estimated new sputum smear-positive tuberculosis cases.

Case notifications represent only a fraction of the true number of cases in a country because the coverage by effective NTPs will be incomplete.

The estimated case detection rate is defined as:

Case detection rate (%) = $\dfrac{\text{Annual new smear-positive notifications (country)}}{\text{Estimated annual new smear-positive incidence (country)}}$

DOTS detection rate refers to case detection under DOTS:

DOTS detection rate (%) = $\dfrac{\text{Annual new smear-positive notifications under DOTS}}{\text{Estimated annual new smear-positive incidence (country)}}$

The case detection rate and DOTS detection rate are identical when a country has a 100% DOTS enrolment rate. Updated estimated incidence for 2001 in this report was provided by WHO, Geneva.

Population with access to DOTS: The country's population that has access to units implementing DOTS.

DOTS Enrolment Rate (%): This indicates a proportion of cases enroled in DOTS out of notified cases.

DOTS enrolment rate (all types) (%) = $\dfrac{\text{Annual notifications of all types under DOTS}}{\text{Total of annual notifications of all types}}$

DOTS enrolment rate (New S+) (%) = $\dfrac{\text{Annual notification of new S+ under DOTS}}{\text{Total of annual notifications of new S+}}$